More praise for
THE NEW GAME PLAN FOR RECOVERY

"This delightful and practical book invites you to discover and recover your sense of self, sense of wonder, and sense of humor. It is filled with enlightening concepts and light-hearted activities to help us move from areas of self-abuse to the richness of self-amuse. This book works!"

> Dr. Joel Goodman
> Director, The HUMOR Project, Inc.

"Foolishness!! Silliness!! Things to avoid, right? Wrong! Tobin and Tom take a playful look at lowering our stress, lightening our hearts and freeing up our soul. A practical, readable and delightful book chock full of actual wisdom traveling in the company of many smiles."

> Steve Allen, Jr., M.D.
> Family physician and humorist

"Within these pages, Tobin and Tom have established a game plan that most anyone can follow, and you don't have to worry about not following the game plan if the other team starts winning, because there is no other team, and the only person who loses is the person who doesn't play."

> Karl Rohnke
> President, Project Adventure, Inc.

"This profound, joyful book proves that it's never too late to have a happy childhood."
Tom Ferguson, M.D.

> Co-author of
> *The Stethoscope Book & Kit*

"Tobin and Tom are two guys who are serious about having fun. This is an upbeat, fun-filled book that not only tells you *why* adults need to be more playful, but actually shows you *how* to do it."

> Matt Weinstein
> Author of *Playfair*

The New Game Plan for Recovery

Rediscovering the Positive Power of Play

Tobin Quereau and
Tom Zimmermann

Illustrations by David Spohn

Ballantine Books
New York

Library of Congress Catalog Card Number: 91-92160
ISBN: 0-345-36566-6

Cover design by Kristine V. Mills
Cover illustration copyright © Laurie Zagon
Text design by Beth Tondreau Design

Manufactured in the United States of America
First Edition: March 1992
10 9 8 7 6 5 4 3 2 1

To my father, Douglass Worthy Quereau,
for teaching me that play is rewarding at any age,
and to my daughter, Jennifer Catherine Quereau,
for reminding me that the time for it is now!

TQ

To my parents, Augie and Rita Zimmermann,
who created my first circle of support, trust, and love,
and had fun all along the way.

TZ

CONTENTS

ACKNOWLEDGMENTS

Our thanks for support, assistance, encouragement, and inspiration must remain inadequate at best. Besides those people mentioned specifically (and sincerely) here, many more have contributed in ways as valuable and important though they remain anonymous. In many instances, the limitations of our memory and a lack of information preclude a more accurate honoring of our benefactors.

We offer our thanks to all of the "unacknowledged contributors" in our lives. For the most part, you know who you are. Please accept our heartfelt appreciation for your gifts to us, and know that we dearly hope you will take some pride in the result of our collaboration. For those ways in which we may not measure up to the value of your contribution, we of course take full responsibility.

Those who have mentored us through their own work, knowingly or not, are generally mentioned as resources at appropriate places in the text. Others to whom we have been indebted over the years include Angeles Arrien, Robert Bly, Joseph Campbell, Jack Canfield, Bill Moyers, Joseph Chilton Pearce, Annie Robinson, Prana and Yamuna, Rosemarie Schultz, and Swami-ji.

Of those many who have helped us on specifically this project, we thank the following:

Claudia Black, Sharon Wegscheider-Cruse, and Joe Cruse for personal and professional inspiration, support, advice, encouragement, friendship, and playful interaction over the years. Phil Orrick for having the audacity to give us our first "gig" and the courage to continue asking us for more. Gary Seidler and Peter Vegso for first inviting us to "go national." Martha Perkins and the Listening Tree crew for putting up with our antics over the years and having faith that we would eventually amount to something. Victoria and Bob Hendricks for the generous and invaluable loan of the computer on which this was written.

For the delightful look, feel, and form of this book we gratefully acknowledge the following people: Cheryl Woodruff, our editor, for her playful insight, unfailing support, and unflapable serenity on the long path to publication; Jeff Doctoroff, assistant editor, for his constant good nature and encouragement while juggling details, deadlines, and occasionally Koosh balls; David Spohn, our illustrator, for his heart-warming depictions of the New Game Plan in action; Laurie Zagon, artist, for sharing her artwork with the world and for bringing the cover of our book to life; Mary Ann Emerson, for her exquisite calligraphy on the Free Child Certificate; Alan Pogue, photographer, for his unique ability to make us finally look good in a photograph.

Tobin personally acknowledges the following people as well:

Jennifer Evans for her consummate skill in bringing the best out of my writing before I was even sure a book was possible. My parents, Douglass and Catherine, and my brothers, Charles and Kent, with whom I have shared a lifetime of play. Tom Zimmermann, my "other brother," whose unfailing optimism, unending sense of humor, and continuing delight in bringing people together has carried me forward on paths I would not have discovered, much less explored, on my own. Also I thank Tom for the creative assistance, inspiration, and impetus for the development of the New Game Plan for Recovery workshops outlined in chapters 6 through 9, and his enthusiastic support for all my efforts in writing about what we do.

Most important, I acknowledge the essential and abiding contribution made by my colleague, partner, and wife, Jeanne Quereau. In ways no one else can know, she has made it possible for me to follow my dreams and find them fulfilled more often than I had ever imagined possible.

Tom personally acknowledges the following people:

My parents, brothers, and sisters, from whom I learned that hard work and enthusiastic play are made for each other. Tobin, my "brother," friend, teacher, and partner in play without whom I could *never* have written this book. He has been an inspiring writer, rewriter, and editor, and a playmaster of ever-ready imagination.

I would also like to acknowledge my life-partner and wife, Ellen Zimmermann, with whom I share play, children, and super synergy. Ellen, I look forward to fun and love forever with you.

Finally, both of us, Tom and Tobin, wish to honor and acknowledge the essential contribution made by *all* who have trusted, risked, and responded so playfully over the years to the New Game Plan for Recovery. We could not have done this without you!

*Play is essential for life. . . . It is not selective,
it is mandatory.*
DR. O. CARL SIMONTON

---

*Play has a tendency to be beautiful. . . . The words we
use to denote the elements of play belong for the most part
to aesthetics, terms with which we try to describe the effects of beauty: tension, poise, balance, contrast, variation, solution, resolution, etc. Play casts a spell over us;
it is ''enchanting,'' ''captivating.'' It is invested with the
noblest qualities we are capable of perceiving in things:
rhythm and harmony.*
JOHAN HUIZINGA

---

*There are some things so serious that
you have to laugh at them.*
NIELS BOHR

On the seashores of endless worlds, children play.
SRI RABINDRANATH TAGORE

INTRODUCTION

Work and play are words used to describe the same thing under differing circumstances.
MARK TWAIN

Tom Zimmermann and I, Tobin Quereau, met in 1980 at an outdoor festival in a park in Austin, Texas. We had each managed to maintain so-called childlike qualities further into adulthood than is generally sanctioned in our society, and when we crossed paths, we sensed an almost tangible connection. Here was someone who understood!

Since we had both been attracted to the New Games movement and had been trained by the New Games Foundation in its fascinating brand of imaginative play, we hit it off immediately.

New Games is a form of play developed in the San Francisco Bay area by a group of innovative players in the early 1970s. As they said in one of their brochures, New Games encourages participation, community, and creativity.

The attitude of New Games players is that *any* game can become a New Game when everyone can play, when the fun is shared by all, when the game changes to fit the players rather than the reverse, when people are brought together in cooperation instead of separated by competition, and when the joy of playing—not the score at the end of the game—is the real purpose for participating. New Games has only three general rules: Play Hard, Play Fair, and Nobody Hurt! (If you still don't know what New Games is, you will after reading part 2 of this book.)

By the time Tom and I got to know each other, the New Games Foundation, which had held trainings and tournaments across the country for years, was winding down and has since gone on to the Great Playground in the Sky. But the spirit of New Games is eternal and continues in various other guises as novices and veteran players have carried the torch into the future.

We owe a debt of inspiration and instruction to all the New Games folks and are committed to carrying on the spark in whatever ways we can.

Tom and I began to get together for fun and, whenever possible, enlarged our playgroup of two by bringing in friends, acquaintances, and other willing playmates. As we gradually began working together in the counseling field as well, and spending more and more time together (we had plenty of free time in those early years of "private" practice), there occurred a phenomenon that has persisted to the present day: People began to have a hard time telling us apart. At that point we knew that we were brothers in practice if not in fact, and we have enjoyed that sort of relationship since then.

As we learned more about the issues of chemical dependency in our role as counselors over the years, we began to understand that its impact was not only on the dependent person but also on all the other family members. As we worked with dependent persons, spouses, parents, and children, we couldn't help but notice the relevance of what we were doing with New Games to the process of recovery for all those affected.

In 1982, for the Annual Summer Institute of what was then the Texas Commission on Alcoholism, in Austin, Texas, we designed the first workshop of the New Game Plan for Recovery. We were overwhelmed and delighted by the enthusiasm, intensity, and energy of the hundred-plus participants during the two evening presentations. We knew then that we had found an audience for what we loved to do.

Over the next year or so, Tom and I each learned much more about the effects of alcoholism in our own families of origin as well as in the families of people in our workshops. It felt like we were coming home.

The story doesn't end there. As we began offering the New Game Plan in a great variety of settings, we saw the importance of what we were doing to those who were *working* in the recovery system. The stress of providing support to those addressing their chemical dependency or co-dependency, whether in treatment centers or in peer support settings, is a heavy burden for anyone to shoulder. The burnout and turnover rates are very high. We realized that finding a natural way to enjoy life to the fullest is as important to those offering help as it is to those seeking it; it is a lesson we often have to remind ourselves of.

All that experience and discovery, and more besides, led up to the writing of this book.

After each of our New Game Plan for Recovery presentations, whether at a conference, in a treatment center, or at a weekend workshop, people would come up to us and say, "Where can I get a copy of what we just did?" We would refer them to some of the sources we had drawn from in developing the material; but that didn't really do the trick. We just had to put it down on paper.

As we got underway with the workshop activities, we

realized that many potential readers would not have access to an already formed group of players, as we did in the workshop. Besides, many valuable outlets for play come in forms and settings that might offer perfect opportunities for solitary play. And not everyone who could use more play in their life would identify with the issue of chemical dependency or co-dependency!

So we developed several chapters on play that could be used not only individually by our readers *whatever* their background and interests but also socially and professionally as well when appropriate for bringing the positive power of play into others' lives.

In part 1 of this book we seek to inspire, encourage, and motivate you to increase the level of play, enjoyment, and fun in your life—including your inner life—and in the lives of those around you. The activities described here are appropriate for inclusion in personal recovery programs, stress management plans, therapy client homework assignments, family enrichment activities, and plain old everyday life.

In part 2 we render as faithfully as we can on paper the play-by-play activities of a typical New Game Plan workshop; some of you may want to use such activities in groups you already participate in or lead, or plan to join. Building play into group activities, treatment programs, church meetings, community picnics, and the like can increase the trust, involvement, interaction, satisfaction, and commitment of all who take part.

Part 3 takes you on an excursion both inwardly and outwardly; you will stretch familiar boundaries and explore the healing potential of play from different perspectives.

In hopes that someday we may have an opportunity to play with you more directly, Tom and I welcome you now to our world and invite you to make it your own.

PART

I

*A Personal
Program of Play*

1

Play and Possibility

There ain't nothin' better than fun.
PENNY GELBER (AGE 6)

Play . . . Peek-a-boo with an infant. Pat-a-cake with a two-year-old. Parks and playgrounds. Sand boxes and sandlots. Evening-time tag and nighttime pillow fights.

Play? That's kid's stuff!

And so it is. Children universally play. In all cultures, in one way or another, children spend as much time as they can—and "Please just one minute more!"—in play. In fact, certain types of play—games of chase and chance, make-believe, rhythm and rhyme—seem to be part of some vast language of pleasure, as familiar to children on any one continent as on another. The words may differ, the images vary, but the action is the same—and so is the attraction.

So what? What does this have to do with you? Probably

3

most people reading this book no longer qualify as children (though there is some doubt about a few of us). But no matter what your present age or stage, there are lessons of great value available to you in the lives of children and, more important, in the life of the child within you.

Scientists are beginning at the most general and all-inclusive levels to explore the possibility that the childlike qualities mankind exhibits, of which play is one of the most prevalent, are the reason we have developed into the beings we are. Ashley Montagu, a noted scientist and writer in the realm of human development and behavior, explains this idea better than we can. The following passage is from his book *Growing Young*:

> The truth about the human species is that in body, spirit, feeling, and conduct we are designed to grow and develop in ways that emphasize rather than minimize childlike traits. We are programed to remain in many ways childlike; we were never intended to grow 'up' into the kind of adults most of us have become. . . .
>
> The retention of juvenile physical traits is one of the major qualities that differentiate human beings from other animals, and when this quality is carried over from physical traits to behavioral patterns, human beings can revolutionize their lives and become for the first time, perhaps, the kinds of creatures their heritage intends them to be—that is, youthful all the days of their lives.
>
> What, precisely, are those traits of childhood behavior that are so valuable and that tend to disappear gradually as human beings grow older? We have only to watch children to see them clearly displayed: Curiosity is one of the most important; imaginativeness; playfulness; open-mindedness; willingness to experiment; flexibility; humor; energy; receptiveness to new ideas;

> *honesty; eagerness to learn; and perhaps the most per-*
> *vasive and the most valuable of all, the need to love.*
> *All normal children, unless they have been corrupted*
> *by their elders, show these qualities every day of their*
> *childhood years.*

If we as individuals wish to draw on the very energy that has brought us so far along in the development of our species, we can look to the lessons the young have to offer us and reawaken that energy in our own life.

That's not as easy as it may sound. For most of us the natural curiosity, creativity, and playfulness of our youth was rather rapidly undermined by certain notions about compliance, competitiveness, and competence that permeate our educational system. One research study found that between the ages of five and seven, when most children enter school, the measurable creativity level drops by 80 percent!

We are taught all too soon to grow up, to act our age, to get to work instead of play. The illusions of adulthood replace the fantasies of childhood and we consider the exchange beneficial. The reality is that we too soon lose the laughter, joy, and eagerness for learning that are the hallmarks of the child. And *that's* for those of us who had it good growing up.

For many others the trouble started much sooner.

Some of us had to grow up even more quickly, to take on responsibilities far beyond those nature intended for young children. In many cases, for example, children who grew up in families with alcoholism, workaholism, physical or sexual abuse, divorce, or chronic illness, the natural tendency toward play was disrupted at even an earlier age than for others and the powerful, positive benefits of play were restricted or distorted to an even greater degree. For them, even the recollection of play seems impossible, much less the recovery of it.

But what's the use anyway in recapturing our past, when growing up is hard enough to do? Who's got time to worry about playing when there's work to be done! Why bother to try?

In a word, one reason is **STRESS**!

Hardly a day goes by without some major publication or some television or radio program highlighting the negative effects of stress on our health, work performance, or relationships. The disease of our time—unrelieved, unproductive, and unmanaged stress—is at the core of many of our greatest losses through illness, broken homes, and broken dreams.

It just so happens, however, that the sources of stress in our lives today are minor compared to what they were as we entered this life. Imagine finding yourself in a completely alien environment, not knowing *any* language, uncertain why you are here, totally dependent on others who may or may not be there when you need them. It's tough enough just visiting a foreign country for a vacation; think how bad our arrival on this planet must have felt to us. No wonder we forgot it so quickly.

But as infants we all made it through while, at the same time, accomplishing the greatest feats of learning we ever manage to achieve: figuring out what our bodies are and how they work; entering into the world in a functional way; creating language; and negotiating the delicate dance of relationships—and all that *before* we reach school age!

So there must be something we knew as kids that we could sure use now. Grace under pressure, serenity in the face of uncertainty, joy in spite of circumstances, and the sense of life as an adventure worth living.

Play isn't all of it. Kids may succeed as much through what they don't know as from what they do. They have society's permission to bend the rules a bit until they learn them. They can say the things we keep under our breath, do the things we wouldn't dare, and let the world go fly a kite if things aren't going their way (*some* of the time, at any rate). And they do have others watching out for them along the way.

But the fact remains that kids handle stress fairly well. They learn and grow with amazing agility. They bounce back with almost uncanny resilience. They live life with incredible intensity. Wouldn't you like to borrow even a bit of their energy?

It can be done. Recent explorations into the power of play as a rejuvenating (notice the reference to juvenile?) healing force in our lives suggest that we may carry *within us* the real source of vibrant, vigorous health.

Norman Cousins' famous experiences in recuperation from major life-threatening diseases centered on his ability to activate his own immune system through a concentrated focus on laughter, playfulness, and joy, among other things. As reported in his last book, *Head First: The Biology of Hope*, Cousins collected extensive evidence from reputable scientific researchers on the connection between mental and emotional states and recovery from illness. Some studies have found that even a smile stimulates the brain's production of endorphins, one of the most potent painkillers ever discovered.

As a result of such studies, there is a whole new branch of medicine, psychoneuroimmunology, which studies the impact of attitudes and expectations on the brain, the endocrine system, and the immune system.

More and more often, treatment plans for such diverse diseases as depression, cancer, and high blood pressure include prescribed doses of relaxation, enjoyment, and play. If play can be helpful in such dire circumstances, should we doubt its value on a daily basis for our overall health and wellness?

And there is more.

For those people who have grown up in stressed, troubled homes, the effects are doubly difficult to manage.

The very strategies they learned as children to help them survive may contribute to their levels of stress as they become adults. What may have worked in the particular context of their family may be limiting in the realities of their adult life.

Indeed, an entire community of people are now forthrightly identifying themselves—adult children of alcoholics, or survivors of sexual abuse, for example—as part of their process of recovery from wounds received early in life. Encouraged by others who have experienced similar problems, they believe that until they recognize the impact of the stress they have struggled with for years, they cannot achieve full satisfaction in their present relationships, work, and leisure activities.

Our life as a child is not simply left behind as we grow older. As William Wordsworth said, "The child is the father of the man." Our experiences within our family of origin shape us in powerful ways as we grow, and as adults we may at times respond to certain situations or people with remarkably childish behaviors.

The popular literature on the subject of growing up in a troubled family has identified the typical roles that children may take on in order to survive: the Hero or Superresponsible Role, the Rebel or Scapegoat Role, the Lost Child or Adjuster Role, and the Clown or Mascot Role.

These roles and others are adopted by children in all families; it is just that in troubled families the roles are more rigid, limiting, and isolating. The range of safe, supported behaviors is much narrower and each child's identity is more directly linked to the role he or she plays than in healthier families.

Such learned behaviors and family patterns interrupt the natural stages of development and form a base for each person's sense of self. They generally persist long into adulthood, even when the circumstances have changed and the roles are no longer needed.

The term "adult child" is descriptive in both of its aspects: As children we may have had to be more grown-up than we would have wanted, and as adults we may feel more like children than we would like anyone else to know.

This very condition has its positive side. In the process of recovery, of revisiting and releasing past traumas endured, we can draw upon the strengths as well as the struggles we knew as children. By discovering the child within each of us, we may be able to bring some of the vitality, energy, excitement, and wonder that are the gifts of the young into the fullness of our adult life.

What's in it for us?

If we are to agree with Ashley Montagu, we find that we have all grown up too far, and some of us too fast as well. We have lost the freshness of youth, the freedom of movement and thought, the pleasure of the sensory world, and the delight of the imaginative ones. As one proverb has it, we grow too soon old, and too late smart.

But there is hope. One characteristic that sets us apart as human beings is our ability to continue learning and growing, all life long.

We *can* once again experience the power of play, *no matter how we feel at the moment.* Tom Robbins, a novelist with a marvelously developed sense of the playful, has put it this way: "It's never too late to have a happy childhood!"

Ashley Montagu's goal (he is in his eighties as we write) is to die as young as he can—as late in life as possible.

Our goal with this book is to help you create, promote, and allow into your life more spontaneity, delight, joy, excitement, curiosity, wonder, and just plain old FUN. *It can be done.* We are going to show you how.

How about it? Will you come out and play?

If at this moment you feel tempted to put down this book in favor of doing the laundry or cleaning out the attic, you are one of those we are writing for. You have already begun the work of self-change by reading this far, and we congratulate you. Don't despair: All those ambivalent, uncomfortable sensations you are now experiencing are to be expected. That's why we start out this program of recovery with an exploration of the barriers between you and play.

Playing with Blocks

For many good reasons, people, especially grown-ups, have a hard time with playing. Just so you don't feel too self-conscious or unique, we decided to talk about some of those reasons right up front.

Everyone plays with blocks.

It is just that the kind of block we are referring to changes as we grow older. The wooden variety does just fine for the youngest of us; but as we increase in skill, sophistication, experience, and age, our blocks become decidedly more abstract, personal, and emotional. What started out as a marvelous medium for creativity is more often associated in later years with the absence of the same. We block our communication, our feelings, and eventually even our arteries. In short, we get stuck.

With awareness, however, we can learn to be compassionate observers of our limitations—without being limited to them out of habit. On occasion we may even move beyond them, and explore new territory.

We now haul out some typical blocks to look at with you. In the process, we think, you'll see pretty clearly that you are among friends who understand what you may be going through. These specific blocks are the result of extensive research conducted over a period of years and compiled in a matter of minutes and in no particular order as we sat in Tom's loft one Sunday afternoon. Feel free to add to them as you see fit.

Block #1: Fear of Loss of Control

Let's face it. Few things seem to bring you as close to being *out of control* as playing does. It just isn't play when you know exactly how things are going to turn out. Playing is almost impossible without learning to let go. Under this heading also come the associated fears: of being vulnerable, not knowing how, being taken advantage of, and the like. Who in their right mind likes to be out of control of a situation? No one we know.

But the problem is not with "play." The problem comes when we confuse the process of play with actually being out of control. For children, play is a primary way of *gaining* control in life.

Play is the process that lets us retain some control in a situation that, were we not playing, could be very scary or even dangerous. Play lets us explore our edges, enlarge our limits, and experience the unacceptable without undue penalty precisely because we *are* still playing. If we don't like the results, we can always take our ball and go home. Suffice it to say that when we play as adults, we often forget who is making the rules.

Block #2: Fear of Looking Foolish

Sometimes, the focus is on "What Will People Think?" rather than on how much control we have in the situation. We have all made fools of ourselves at some point in our lives. Sometime when we least expected it, someone somewhere zapped us—with devastating results that we have yet to overcome. Nothing hurts in quite the same way.

Whatever its sources, the problem here is one of *trust*. We have lost our sense of who makes a good playmate and who doesn't. A result of this confusion is that we lose the ability to play even if everyone else *is* playing. What if someone should make fun *of* us instead of *with* us? Horrors! And if we can't trust them, how can we trust ourselves?

Well, the fact is, there will always be times when we get zapped by someone else. And we may well have been through some particularly gruesome incidents when we were playing and someone else was not. But the answer is not to give up playing. How about chucking those creeps instead?

Block #3: Fear of Failure

Now this is a biggie. It is tied quite closely with the predominant ethic in our social interaction: competition. How many times have you dropped the ball, lost the point, run the wrong way, tripped over your own foot? Have you ever felt like crawling under the grass so no one could see? Welcome to the world of ADULT PLAY. "Winning isn't everything, it's the only thing." Or, "No one asks who came in second!" You know the routine. Heaven forbid if the game should be lost because of YOU. And, of course, we *know* that everything depends on you. Maybe you should just give up!

Actually, this may be a question of *over-responsibility*. For some, the fear of failure is so great because something or someone had made them feel, early in life, that everything depended on them. *If they didn't do it, no one else would!* (And "it" may have been a vitally important task.) For others, the smallest failure turned out to be a catastrophe in the eyes of someone else in a person's life—someone too important to ignore. Again, it's part of growing up too soon.

Fortunately, until they are "corrupted by their elders," kids don't see it that way. The paramount principle of play is to have fun! If things aren't going their way, then they change the game. Kids even have fun constructing the most magnificent failures possible. Anything is fair game for a fun-loving five-year-old. . . .

Block #4: Acting Your Age

The further we go, the more we come back to this basic objection. All of this "play stuff" runs counter to proper behavior for ADULTS. You see, as ADULTS we know that you have to work for what you want, that money doesn't grow on trees, that the "good things" in life don't come cheap, and that you don't get ahead by "messing around." After all, we have our reputations to consider.

Even the ADULT world of recreation has its own rules and regulations. We practice, exercise, discipline ourselves, invest in equipment, join leagues, clubs, and tournaments. And win, lose, or draw, we sure as hell keep score! The biggest problem with all of this is that it isn't much different from what we do for a living most days of the week. In the face of life's lessons, we have a hard time letting go of our hard-won "maturity." It's a tough world out there and we'd better stay on our toes every minute!

It *is* difficult to believe that there may be another way. But think again of the world we each entered in the beginning. With no clear sense of where we were, what we were doing here, or how we would get our needs met, we struggled to make sense out of things.

By paying attention to the moment more than to the past or the future, by tuning in to how we felt without undue judgment, by expressing ourselves as clearly and directly as we could, and by playing with the world whenever and wherever we could, we made it through trials and tribulations none of us would willingly take on today.

It's true that we had some help, some of us more than others. But the fact remains that we played our way into existence from the very beginning. If we can just learn to keep on playing as we grow older, maybe we'll find just as much mystery and magic, renewal and reward in the present and the future as we did in the distant past.

Block #5: I Don't Have the Time

O.K., O.K., so I believe you already! But I've got work to do. There's the house to clean and the taxes to file and the New Year's letter to all of our friends to write. I'd love to have the time to play around, but there's just too much going on, and . . .

That's precisely what we said to ourselves for the five years we spent discussing whether, whither, and when to write this book. Of course it wasn't so much that we didn't have the time—no one does. It was that we weren't *taking* the time for something we kept saying was important to us and might be important to others as well.

It's a matter of *choice*. We can continue to talk about what we want while acting in direct contradiction to that desire, or we can start finding creative ways to bring play, pleasure, and positive feelings into our life even as we do what needs to be done.

Play is an attitude as much as an action. We have to value its benefits and rewards in order to invest our time and energy in it. The choice is not so much for this *or* that, but for ourselves. And we deserve it!

Control, trust, over-responsibility, "acting" our age, avoidance of feelings, choices—these and other issues are at the heart of how we block ourselves from growing, changing, and enjoying life. We are all subject to blocks, some of us more than others, some in different ways than others. The trick is to avoid judging ourselves too harshly because of them. If we can keep that tendency at bay, ultimately we can learn to play even with our blocks—

letting go a bit more each day, taking appropriate responsibility for our well-being, trusting that we can act as young as we feel, and finding time for the joys as well as the stresses of life.

Sounds like a big order? It is. Fortunately we knew a lot about how to handle it at least once in the past, and we can relearn those skills. Let's take a look at what the experts in stress management have to offer us.

Child's Play

What exactly is child's play? In our experience, both of growing up and of observing children of all ages at play, we have noted several characteristics of play that are worth highlighting.

Play, for example, seems to be more about *process* than product. The forts we built were never "finished," the wars we fought never really "won." The outcome was not as critical as the engagement—even winning was just an opening for "one more game!" The accomplishment achieved was not as satisfying as the accomplishing of it, and even failure held a sense of promise more than of finality. Indeed, total mastery meant boredom as much as anything else.

This brings up the sense of *challenge* that seemed to permeate the experience of play when we were children. In some cases more pronounced—remember the exquisite shiver of fear as one hid from approaching footsteps; the last desperate leap across the "safe" line before being tagged—in other cases more subdued—as in playing house or "just pretend"—however it occurred, there was a certain element of tension, of intensity in play that was followed, when all went well, by a euphoric relaxation and resolution that suited everyone (or the game was changed).

A third essential aspect of play was the sense of *freedom*

in the play world that was all too lacking in other realms. In play all things were possible. Molehills *became* mountains. Trees flew into space. Bad guys were vanquished (unless you were on their side) and you never had to be killed except by choice. Time and space were no barriers until it was time for supper or bed. You could do anything you wanted to—as long as you could convince the others to go along with your game plan.

The problem was, play was basically a *voluntary* activity and "ol' Larry" wouldn't play unless he wanted to. Samuel Clemens writing as Mark Twain once had Tom Sawyer say, "Work consists of whatever a body is obliged to do. . . . Play consists of whatever a body is not obliged to do." That accounts in part for the exhaustive discussions of "Whaddaya wanna do?" They seemed to take up the greater part of the available playtime. Beyond that the only real restrictions were the *rules*—they were important in order to maintain the challenge. But then one could always "play" with the rules, too.

Child's play, you see, mostly takes place in the world of the *imagination*. While ADULT play is often limited to the boundaries of the "real" world, children create worlds as needed, import miracles on demand, soar beyond all limits as a matter of course, and sacrifice nothing that can't be reconstituted on the spot (or as soon as the other person turns his or her back). Children play not to strengthen their bodies, to reduce their stress, to clinch a deal, or to make a buck. Children play *because it feels good*! It's fun!

They make a world in which they are in control, in which they are the creators. It is a world in which danger lurks and power pervades, fear excites and disaster threatens. It is engagement in life under their own terms. And if things don't work out the way they want, they play something else!

Wait, you say. *No wonder we adults don't play like that—*

it's dangerous! The REAL world doesn't work that way. It's amazing that kids survive to be adults, with that attitude. Can you imagine what would happen if people were free to quit their jobs or throw away their bills anytime things weren't going the right way?

We know, you're perfectly right, the ADULT REAL WORLD isn't that way. In the ADULT REAL WORLD we must pay taxes unless we are too rich, pay insurance unless we are too poor, and do both if we are stuck in the middle. In the ADULT REAL WORLD vacations end, Mondays come too soon, and Fridays not soon enough. In the ADULT REAL WORLD the clocks run all of the time, we get tired when we are active, we grow old, suffer, and die before we are ready.

But it doesn't have to be that way *all* the time. As adults we *can* recover some measure of the magic and mystery, joy and rejuvenation that is our heritage and our promise. In full control of our faculties and finances, with sound minds and healthy bodies, we can rediscover how to play in the rewarding, renewing way our children do. We can even love it, too.

There is much more that could be said, but let's just summarize by saying *Play is a voluntary activity that is at once invigorating and relaxing, challenging and rewarding, unpredictable yet unthreatening; and above all it is a process we enjoy.*

Play brings us into "present time"; it teaches us flexibility and responsiveness; it encourages creativity and inventiveness. It stimulates body, mind, and spirit and increases their integration and coordination. In short, it revitalizes us and brings us in contact with that intrinsic joy of living so essential to learning and growth.

By watching the lives of children—and our own "inner child"—we can learn that most powerful of lessons, *that life can be its own reward.*

Perhaps play isn't just for kids. Perhaps we set it aside

all too easily for our own good. Perhaps our health and well-being are as well served by appropriate play as by appropriate diet, exercise, work, rest, and relationships.

How do *you* play? How often? How long? Imagine yourself playing in some new and satisfying way starting today. Can you do it?

It's a possibility.

2

It's Never Too Late

What then is the right way of living?
Life must be lived as play. . . .
PLATO

The most eloquent descriptions of play and its benefits for the health and happiness of all humankind are worth nothing if they don't lead to action.

The proof is in the playing.

While there is a necessary and valuable place for theories and philosophies of play, our goal is much more basic (and perhaps more difficult). We would like to help you change your *behavior* toward play.

Thoughts and ideas, being in the realm of the mind, are not bound by time and space. Given the right information or insight, we can change our minds instantaneously. Our bodies, however, our hearts and hands, are of a different dimension. They move to different rhythms and respond in their own time. Changing behavior, therefore, is of necessity a slower process, one accompanied by unfamiliar and sometimes uncomfortable feelings as we grow into new ways of being.

But our head, heart, and hands are intimately connected, and we *can* initiate change from any one of them. We subscribe to that famous dictum, seeing is believing—and find it almost as often true in reverse. When we believe something is possible we are more likely to find ourselves doing it and when we find ourselves doing something, we are more likely to believe it is possible.

If you are one of the many adults who don't think play is an entirely legitimate pastime, we encourage you to adopt the strategy employed by most master players from two-year-olds on up—make-believe!

Fake it until you make it.

Find out for yourself just how valuable a playful attitude and experience can be in your life. In this chapter we will outline some activities that have helped thousands of people stimulate their creativity, maximize their sense of wonder, delight, and joy, and increase their skill as first class FUN-raisers.

We need to know where we are in order to begin to change, however, so we will recommend that before we go any further you take your own personal PDQ. Just write what you come up with right here after this colon:

What? You don't know what a PDQ is? Sorry, we should have introduced it more carefully. Your PDQ is your Play Development Quotient. It is the number from 1 to 100 that represents for you right now how *you* feel about the amount and quality of play in your life.

For example, a 1 would be shorthand for: I don't know what play is, I don't think I have ever indulged in it on purpose, and if I did any of it by accident I would quit as soon as I figured out what I was doing so that I could get back to work (or at least back to worrying about work).

If you are seriously considering putting down a 1 we would like to congratulate you for making it this far and to warn you it doesn't get any easier as you continue in the New Game Plan for Recovery. What you are about to do will constitute some of the toughest work you will ever have to do. We will understand if the going gets too tough for you and you decide to give up—temporarily—and take a rest from the program.

A 100, on the other hand, is for someone who has never quite quit playing from day one. If you play in some way every day and can think of a hundred more ways you could play if you just had the time, you may be a natural 100 in your PDQ. In such a case, please write to us as soon as possible and let us know all you know about play so we can generate more material for our sequel to the New Game Plan.

Oh yes, we don't allow anyone to pick 50. Those of you who just winced are candidates for designation as "Mugwumps." You put your "mug" on one side of an issue, and your "wump" on the other. We want you to make a definitive statement about how you feel right now about play. Would you consider a 49 or a 51?

At any rate, we *do* want you to pause long enough here to come up with your best intuitive assessment of your Play Development Quotient. We will be referring to it again in the future; and we're betting that if you put it on record now, you'll be amazed later on to see how far you've come.

Our first real assignment in this practicum on play is to do some in-depth research on the topic. Each of us has been at some point in the past a master in the art of play. As hard as it may be to believe, each of us was a child once. And because the business of children is play, some-where back there in the dusty past we must have spent as much time as possible in the pursuit of play.

The qualifying word "possible" is important here. We

are not saying that kids do nothing but play. Eating, sleeping, learning the hard way, and arguing with their parents and siblings take up a fair share of the day. And, for many, the environment they grow up in is not conducive to much overt activity of a playful quality.

For some former children, the very recollection of a childhood at all, much less the playful part, is still an impossibility. That doesn't mean they did not have experiences of play that they can recover eventually, as they reclaim their childhood and the child that remains within them. It just may be that they will have to allow themselves more time and attention on the subject in order to reap the benefits.

But let's get started. This research assignment we mentioned is one we call:

Guided Replay

We are going to join you on a journey back through your positive experiences of play. You can share with others the results of this process; in fact the benefits will be greater for your doing so. But the journey itself requires a quiet space and some time to yourself without interruption.

You can even record the instructions (they're coming right up) on a tape recorder with gentle music in the background. Leave some time between questions for you to recall specific experiences, and then sit back and give yourself the gift of revisiting some magical moments of your youth.

Please make yourself comfortable and take a moment to notice the rhythm and depth of your breathing. . . . We will be taking you back to some of your earliest experiences of play.

If along the way you find yourself recalling experiences

that were anything but positive, just relax, acknowledgethat those things happened too, and then go back to searching for the times when you felt good, had fun, were rejuvenated and renewed by your play. If you can't seem to remember any positive experiences of play, don't despair. For many people this exercise needs to be repeated several times before they begin to recover their playful times. In these cases it can be especially helpful to discuss play with others. The examples of play they recall can help bring back memories of your own.

To begin, take another deep, slow breath, gently close your eyes, and imagine yourself standing in front of the childhood home in which you remember growing up. You may be any age in the time you're recalling, but whatever house, apartment, farm, or building you actually recollect from your childhood is what we are looking for. Remember what it looked like from in front.

What were the surroundings like?

What was next to it on either side?

Now go up to the front door in your imagination and go inside. Take us with you to your room. . . . Stand in the doorway for a moment and look around.

What do you remember about the walls? What was on them?

What was the furniture like?

Where did you sleep and where were your toys kept (when they weren't all over the floor)?

What were your favorite toys?

Did you share your room with a brother or sister?

What did the two (or more) of you do for fun when you had the time to play?

How did you amuse yourself when you were all alone?

Who were your imaginary friends?

Who were your living, breathing friends?

Did you have a pet to play with?

What were your favorite games, "pretends," and pastimes?

Where did you most enjoy playing in your home?

Where did you run to on a Saturday morning in springtime when the weather was just right and your friends were available to play with?

What did you do for fun down at the corner vacant lot . . . over in the school yard . . . or down by the culvert or creek?

Where did you build your forts, clubs, and tree houses?

Where were your hideouts? (We'll keep the secret!)

What did you play on hot summer afternoons when the street burned your feet and even the crickets had sense enough to stay indoors?

Where did you go and what did you do when the fall rains came and flooded the streets with rushing water and bits of broken twigs and leaves?

What games did you play as evening fell and the darkening sky outlined the trees or the cityscape in deep velvety blue?

How did you spend the brief, cold days of winter when the wind whistled between tree-limbs and through layers of clothing almost as if they weren't there?

In all these seasons and settings—with family and friends, with pets, and all by yourself—you played as a child. With words, wishes, people, and playthings you created a make-believe world where sense and nonsense were deliciously swirled into a treat unmatched in "real" life.

Let yourself now re-experience the sounds and sensations you knew then. As though in a movie you direct and produce, at all the ages and stages you can recall, take all the time you need now to fully recover your own unique and powerfully positive experience of play. . . .

There is no need to rush on with the reading. We will still be here when you return.

When you are ready, bring with you the memories you have uncovered of your experience of play as you gradually stretch, take a deep breath, and slowly open your eyes, feeling rested, relaxed, and alert.

Now (you *have* finished the first assignment, haven't you?) go tell someone you care about what you learned on your journey back. It is even better when they too reveal some of the things they did as a child. We bet that there are more than a couple of ways in which the two of you shared the same activities and interests, actions and interactions. They can probably remind you of a few you had even forgotten.

This particular process of remembering and relating is especially good for bringing together generations of players: parents and kids, grandparents and grandchildren. We would never think of turning it into a school research assignment (though someone *else* might . . .).

We would like to add a word here for those who are perhaps feeling depressed and frustrated by their inability to recapture anything remotely positive. You are our *most* important audience. You, through no fault of your own, may have suffered deprivation, difficulty, and disruption no child should have to endure. But you have endured. You are a survivor. Your pain is a measure of just how bad it was.

We want you to know, however, that in our experience even the most troubled childhood contains moments of pleasure, hours of fun, periods of playful delight. You may not find them now, but we believe they *are* there. And, in any case, the child within you is still available to help you create *from this moment on* what you may not have had much of then.

IT'S NEVER TOO LATE TO HAVE A HAPPY CHILDHOOD!

You may just need more support, encouragement, and practice than some. Be sure to give yourself now what others couldn't give you back then.

The reason for all this ''research'' is to take advantage of two facts: We have all had the experience of play before, and experience is (sometimes) the best teacher. Now that you have some contact with what it felt like to be a player, let that unique set of sensations guide you as you begin to build your repertoire of present-time play.

Becoming playful is really more a process of awakening your Inner Child than it is a requirement for learning something for the first time. We want you to take advantage of your years of expertise.

Your Personal Play Journal

In order that you take full advantage of the research program we are advocating now and of the ensuing course in the art of play, we suggest Step Two in the New Game Plan for Recovery. Your assignment is to visit your local toy store, stationery store, or department store and buy your Personal Play Journal. You might want to find one of those special diaries with lock and key that you can hide away in a secret place.

Your recollections and impressions from the Guided Replay, as detailed as you wish to make them, can be an ideal opening entry in this journal (which you can dedicate to your Inner Child). We will be making many more recommendations, assignments, and the like as we take you through the New Game Plan; and having an ongoing record of the changes and challenges you undergo will be your priceless gift to yourself and your Inner Child. You both deserve it.

Just don't forget to talk to someone else about your play life, too, after you have written down what you remembered. You can always make additions as you get the benefit of responses from others.

And speaking of play life, we would like to direct your attention to the present as well as the past. This brings us to Step Three in the New Game Plan for Recovery:

Assessing Your Laugh Life

Step Three involves creating your very own Fun List. It is a simple process: You list the fifteen things you do for fun in your life. Yes, we said fifteen. No, it is not sufficient to "think about" the fifteen things, you have to write them down. From one to fifteen. Now. (We even provide the paper!)

My Fun List

1. _____

2. _____

3. _____

4. _____

5. _____

6. _____

7. _____

8. _____

9. _____

10. _____

11. _____

12. _____

13. _____

14. _____

15. _____

We know, you don't have a pen, it is out of ink, you'll come back to this later, you did this once before (you think). All right, we'll give you an option. You can write down fifteen reasons why you *can't* write down the fifteen ways you have fun in your life. That could be fun!

If you are in a total panic by now trying to come up with fifteen ways you have fun in your life, we will give you some pointers. Consider the following suggestions and see if they shake something loose:

What do you do primarily because it feels good? (Remember, this is your own private list; you can put down whatever you want.)

Beginning with getting up in the morning, go through a typical day and recall the things that you look forward to with anticipation. Include the evening and night as well.

Move through your house in your imagination, room by room, and think of the things that are fun in each location. Now, add the yard and the neighborhood to your survey.

Do the same with the places you go to frequently. Could there be anything fun about work, for example?

What about after work, on weekends, on vacations, at different seasons of the year?

Think about those people you like to have fun with. What do you enjoy doing with them?

What about those things you do infrequently?

If you haven't been able to come up with fifteen yet, that may have as much to do with how you define fun as it does with your actual behavior. Try not to assume what others (including us) might count as playful. You have the right to enjoy life in your own unique ways. Even if the activities that come to mind don't seem like much, put down at least fifteen things on your list that you do now for fun (even if making lists isn't one of them).

For those who are *really* interested in increasing the enjoyment in their lives, we have advanced-level fun lists. (There is plenty of room in your Personal Play Journal for these next two lists.) The first is fairly simple, since we just went through the Guided Replay. It's called the *Used-To-Do Fun List*. It is a list of fifteen things you used to do for fun. It can be from any time in your life that seems interesting, but try to include some from recent times as well as ancient ones. The same guidelines can apply.

Then there is the *Wanna-Do Fun List*. This one includes (you guessed it) fifteen things you have always wanted to do for fun, but for one reason or another have never gotten around to trying out. Let yourself go on this one. Money is no object. Time is no barrier. Health is . . . Well, it's O.K. to risk breaking your neck if that risk is only on your list. Be sure to take care of yourself when it comes to actually trying these things out!

Once you have your list (or lists) complete, take a look to see how many and which ones you do regularly. (Remember, regularity is a sign of good health!) Which ones do you experience less frequently? Is that how you want it to be?

How many do you do by yourself? How many with friends? Ideally you will find a balance between the two extremes so that you are able to find enjoyment in either situation.

Check to make sure you don't price yourself out of entertainment by always having to pay for your fun. On the other hand, be sure to value yourself enough to plunk down some solid change every now and then, when you have it to spend, to have a special time.

Finally, make your list long enough *(you mean forty-five items isn't enough?)* to insure that at any moment of the day or night, when you least expect it, you can find something fun to do if the opportunity presents itself. Then be sure that it presents itself on a regular—daily?—basis.

Now why don't you stop here and actually go back to *do* this silly exercise before we move on to something really tough, like . . .

Finding a Playmate

We don't need others to play with. There are endless ways we can enjoy ourselves when we are alone. But when we are just starting out to become childlike again, it can definitely help to have one or more companions join us along the way.

Therefore, we now need to investigate who (and how many) you are going to tap for the signal honor of Playmate Extraordinaire!

Not all of your friends will be good playmates for all types of play. That is why it's useful to sit down with a piece of paper (are you getting the hint? Assignment Number Four!) to list those people you have played with, play with now, or would like to play with.

Then think about which kinds of play each of those people would most be suited for. (See why you should have done your Fun List?) Not everyone gets a bang out of all-night Monopoly binges, for example. The ones who don't may, however, be magnificent flyers of kites. Ice skaters may not be the swiftest skiers, if you get our drift. In any case, here is where you identify the people who can be your partners in play.

My Play Community

PLAYMATES   ACTIVITIES

_____   _____

_____   _____

_____   _____

_____   _____

If, upon staring at the blank page in front of you, not a single name leaps into view, we have stumbled on one of the primary reasons you may not play as much or as often as you would like. In such a case the first game you will need to play is a modified form of Hide-and-Seek. You and your future playmates have been hiding from each other entirely too long and it is high time to do some first-class seeking!

We suggest you start slowly and build up your endurance by finding one new playmate per month, varying your choice as appropriate until you can count on at least five good, high quality playmates with whom you can attempt the rather rigorous program of play we are about to outline. Do remember to let your own sense of timing and choice be the guide. And remember, not all good playmates are identifiable at a distance.

One further note: Don't limit yourself to persons entirely of the same sex, background, or age. Many of our best players are children and some of our most experienced ones are grandparents.

How does all of this look to you so far? Surprised? Encouraged? Depressed? Don't despair, in order to assist you in expanding your repertoire of play, we will also give you the following:

Principles, Practices, and Prescriptions for Play

Principle #1: Play is not for real (but it is real fun!)

When you want to create more fun in your life let yourself go! Check out of this world every now and then and visit one where things *do* turn out the way you want. Take along some friends. Remember, figuring out what you want to do can be as much fun as doing what you figure out. Be less like you usually are than you've ever been before. Then be more like you've always been than you ever dared to be. Either way, it's all for fun. Pretend to be an adult. Kid around. Do something for no particular reason. Quit when you feel like it. Create a space where nothing can go "wrong" so that it doesn't matter if everything does.

Principle #2: When you can do so safely, suspend judgment (and fear of judgment) in favor of fun.

Take some clay, paint, or a musical instrument and practice doing something sloppily. See how it feels. Feel how it sounds. Tell yourself to find something new and unexpected in the results. Be awkward. Use your untrained hand, the wrong tools, close your eyes. Try as hard as you can to do nothing in particular. Write a poem, sing a song. Expand your range of possibilities. Explore. Express yourself. Then throw away what you don't like with no regrets. No one has to know how it all turned out. But then, if you really want some laughs, trade results with a trusted friend who is equally inhibited or uninhibited. Failures can be fun! And try not to be too upset if, by mistake, you discover a great new way of doing something.

Principle #3: Put process before product.

Even in traditional games you can pay more attention to the process than to the outcome. Stay in the moment as you swing, roll, throw, shoot, or move. Let the score go or play to the losing point, replay it, and see how long you can keep the game going. In personal and artistic activities, let yourself be guided by what feels good, not by what you are "supposed" to be drawing, making, singing, or producing. Break the "rules." Make up new ones. Forget them. Forget yourself!

Principle #4: Put some imagination into your challenges.

New Games are delightful examples of the power of pretend, so read the rest of this book, find some friends to play with, and be a kid again. (Remember, suspend judgment in favor of fun.) Spice up whatever you are doing with a bit of make-believe. A little imagination can go a long way.

When you need some new energy to get you through the same old routine, or when you meet a tough assignment head on, use some magic. Don't just cook another meal. Pretend you are a seven-year-old loose in the most realistic playhouse you could imagine, playing with fire, making pies, full of wonder. Or see yourself as a famous French chef whipping up an evening treat for the Baron and Baroness de Lostchild.

Got a tough problem at work? Pretend to be the person you admire the most. How would she or he handle it? Play it all out in your imagination, get excited about your success. Then do it that way for real.

Principle #5:
Do it. . . . . .differently!

Break up your routines in a systematic way. Whenever you think about it, change something. Brush your teeth with the other hand (you may still use a brush if you wish). Towel off in a new way. Put on and tie the other shoe first. Take a new route to work. Be quiet when you would usually speak. Speak up when you least expect it. Read a magazine from back to front. Take a risk—give it back if it's too big. Reward yourself for no special reason. Do the same for someone else. Accept a compliment without flinching—flinch when no one else is around.

Adapt. Modify. Magnify. Minify. Substitute. Rearrange. Reverse. Combine. Surprise yourself with your creativity. And, on occasion, forget to be serious when you re-enter the ADULT REAL WORLD.

Does that give you a few ideas? This isn't an exhaustive list (unless, of course, you choose to do everything in the same day). We trust you can begin to generate your own approaches to bringing more playfulness into your life. Just remember, ideas without action are like bets you never place. You may stay safe, but you're never really in the game either. . . .

Put these principles into practice over a period of time and pay attention to the results. If it feels good, great! Most likely it will also feel unfamiliar, a bit uncomfortable, or even unsettling. Our habits are hard losers in the process of change. But you deserve some fun in your life.

Delight, joy, spontaneity, energy, laughter, and just plain old fun are our birthright as much as anything else the universe has to offer. It is *our* responsibility to insure their presence in our life.

IT'S NEVER TOO LATE. . . .

101 Ways to Have Fun

O.K., so we didn't tell you sooner. You should have known the answers would be in the back of the chapter. Didn't you go to school?

Actually, we know that 90 percent of those who read this book will *not* do the assignments at the time they are assigned. So as a stimulus for getting down to it, we have decided to offer a sample fun list *as a starting point*! Who said we were harsh and demanding? Consider these as a few options for creating your own personal plan of action.

We will start with the ABC's of having fun.

1. arts and crafts shows
2. building bonfires
3. camping out
4. driving in the country
5. exploring new toy stores
6. flying paper airplanes
7. getting a massage
8. hot baths (or tubs)
9. interdigitation (holding hands)
10. junkyard junkets
11. kite flying
12. lying in the shade at the beach
13. midnight swims
14. noontime naps
15. old-time movies
16. petting a pet
17. quiet walks in the snow
18. rock collecting
19. skipping rocks
20. time for reading
21. unexpected surprises

22. vegetable gardening
23. whooping it up
24. Xmas carolling
25. yo-yos
26. zooming down a ski slope

Would you believe "fun in the four seasons?"

WINTER

27. snow ball fights
28. ice skating
29. sleigh rides
30. hot chocolate with whipped cream
31. a fire in the fireplace
32. sledding
33. saunas
34. snow sculptures
35. collecting snowflakes

SPRING

36. hikes in the mountains
37. walking in the rain
38. going to the park
39. visiting a farm
40. canoeing on a river
41. playing volleyball
42. sitting on a porch swing
43. exploring a town off the beaten path
44. backyard cookouts with friends

SUMMER

45. making music
46. poolside parties
47. swimming in a lake
48. admiring boats at a marina
49. seeing a funny movie

50. making sand castles
51. stomping on sand castles
52. taking a child to a magic show
53. late-night talks on the front porch

Fall

54. charades
55. disc golf
56. roller skating
57. roasting marshmallows
58. visits to art galleries
59. guided tours of well-lit caves
60. catching fireflies (and letting them go)
61. fooling around with friends
62. collecting driftwood
63. visiting museums
64. sailboat rides
65. daydreaming
66. hayrides

Anytime

67. naps
68. traveling to some place new
69. going to the theater
70. staying up late
71. sleeping late
72. hobbies
73. going to a party with friends
74. dressing up
75. dressing down
76. amusement parks
77. carnival rides
78. birthday parties
79. collecting things
80. flea markets
81. first-run movies

82. holidays
83. vacations
84. dancing
85. participating in sports
86. spectating
87. watching TV
88. video movies
89. going on picnics
90. pretending
91. goofing off
92. fishing
93. eating out
94. people-watching in the park
95. messing around
96. telling stories to kids
97. board games with buddies
98. watching a sunset
99. playing with babies
100. collecting seashells
101. making wish lists

Now, your mission, should you choose to accept it, is to finish coming up with your *own* fun list, one that reflects ways *you* like to enjoy yourself. It must be *at least* 15 items long. It can be longer.

Then, you are encouraged to pick at least one fun thing per day from the list to *DO!* (That is why having a longer fun list has its advantages; going hang gliding every day could get old after a while.)

For those of you who are still having problems coming up with ideas on how to have more fun, we will refer you to a master fun-list maker, Barbara Ann Kipfer. Her book is entitled *14,000 Things To Be Happy About*, and we will leave it up to you to figure out what it all includes.

Whatever *you* do, have fun with it!

3

Freeing Your Inner Child

*In the true man there is a child concealed—
who wants to play.*
NIETZSCHE

W e trust that something we have shared with you
so far (and, we hope, you will share with others)
has been of value. If so, we have the beginning of a relationship. After all, you *are* still reading! The hours we
have spent in various play communities have certainly
been of great value to *us*. What is most impressive to us
is the powerful sense of awakened energy that radiates
from those who have been through the experience of the
New Game Plan for Recovery and come up to us afterward asking for more.

We would love to take full credit for such amazing
transformations, and we are delighted to accept any
handshakes or hugs that come our way, but the truth is

that we are *not* the source of that warmth and fire. At best we are catalysts for a reaction that rests potentially within each of us. Each one who taps into the power of play is in some way opening up to the positive, creative energy of their own Inner Child.

It doesn't happen so quickly for all; for some it is months or years away. But, once felt, the experience is hard to ignore and the implications go far beyond the reach of the so-called rational mind to suggest that perhaps, just perhaps, there is more to life than we know. The possibility of inviting the wonder, spontaneity, feeling, and fervor of the child into our adult life may seem to be just an unlikely fantasy—but then children are perfectly at home with fantasy.

In this chapter we would like to play matchmakers for a bit. We would like to help you begin or strengthen a relationship with that child within you so that you "both" can benefit.

We use this model of an Inner Child knowing full well that it is *only* a model. Who knows what really describes the marvelously complex nature of a human being? But the use of metaphor and imagery is a powerful tool that children master for growth and learning, and perhaps we too can learn from it.

The potential for self-healing is immense, as evidenced by the popularity and impact of the work of Dr. Charles Whitfield, John Bradshaw, and others. In any case, the image of the Inner Child is compelling and the interaction can be surprising when we relax and let our creative imagination lead the way.

Many who come to play with us report that they have *no* recollection of their childhood to speak of. On activities such as the Guided Replay, they come up frustratingly empty of memories. Others have access to their childhood, but only to the most tragic or problem-laden parts. To suggest they revisit those years is to directly reverse what they have been trying to do for decades. Some adults have never quite felt they graduated from childhood in the first place, feeling all too inadequate and unsure beneath their mask of maturity.

There are those, however, who *have* managed to maintain a balance between growing older and growing young. They are the ones who probably were a part of the proverbial "healthy" family and who seem to have no real difficulty integrating a sense of playfulness and joy into their daily life.

Everyone can benefit from a stronger relationship with the childlike qualities within them. Whether the focus is recovery or discovery, healing or revealing, the path to the child within holds promise of growth and change.

The process is one of making contact and communicating with, and committing ourselves to care for, our Inner Child. It is creating in our inner life the nourishing relationship with our own self that helps us to flourish in the outer world.

Making Contact

Art, imagery, and metaphor have been a road to the inner life for as long as we have been human. Through shape and color, poetry and dance and song, for thousands of years we have called one another to the world within the world.

Our creative imagination, that faculty so marvelously managed even by the youngest of us, has as long a history in the human experience as the more rational aspect of our consciousness, possibly longer. Such "stuff as dreams are made on" is part of the lives of us all, even if we aren't always comfortable with it in the light of day.

Tapping into that creative imagination may be a means to making contact with the child energy within us and initiating a relationship that can renew us all. This next exercise, while similar to the Guided Replay we described earlier in the book, is unique in a fundamental way. Both employ a state of physical and mental relaxation, but the goals are different.

In the Guided Replay the intent is to assist participants in recovering the memories of positive play experiences they had as a child. In the visualizations we are about to share, the goal is to give shape and form, energy and sound to the experience of *being* a child.

For this process, we recommend that you make your own tape recording of the visualization instructions provided below, or find a friend who is willing to assist you as you go through the experience. As with any set of instructions, you are encouraged to use them as suggestions only; anytime you feel a need to adjust or change the focus or follow your own lead, please do so. The very purpose of the instructions is to activate *your* creative imagination.

If you anticipate any discomfort or difficulty, we encourage you to enlist the aid of someone who is experienced in imagery work. A trusted companion can be a valuable asset as you get in touch with your inner life.

The purpose of this visualization is to contact your Inner Child as you experience him or her *now*, not to replay all of your experiences as a child. We are *not* searching here for the "historical" child—the one who went through what you went through growing up. (That is an important piece of work that some people choose to do in a support group or therapy setting, and one that can be an important part of a recovery program. John Bradshaw in his new book *Homecoming* outlines how he works with people in this powerful process of healing the wounded child. That is different from what we are suggesting here, however.)

In this situation we are seeking to contact another level of the Inner Child, the one that came with us into this world. We want to help you reconnect with the positive, powerful, pure energy of the child within you; that entity exists apart from and beyond the impact of external events. John Bradshaw calls this the Wonder Child.

This is a search for our personal source of creativity, spontaneity, and delight in the world, for the *energy* rather than the experiences we knew as a child.

So if uncomfortable material from the past comes up, let it go by rather than focusing on it. Pay attention to your *immediate* experience of your Inner Child and the feelings you have as a result. If things do become too uncomfortable, you can always shift your attention to your current surroundings and bring your awareness back to the present moment; do so if and when you feel the need. Taking good care of yourself is not separable from taking care of your Inner Child.

For now find a quiet place where you feel comfortable and safe. Notice your surroundings, then let them go. . . . Be aware of your breathing, then let it take care of itself. . . . Make your body comfortable, and relax. . . .

In the next few minutes you are going to meet a part of yourself that you may not have contacted for a while. You are going on a journey of exploration that will be an opportunity for learning, discovery, and growth.

Closing your eyes, imagine yourself standing at the edge of a playground in a lovely park. Notice the lush vegetation and savor the scents from the blooming plants nearby. . . . Feel the warmth of the sun against your face and the soft grass beneath your feet as you stand and watch. . . . Listen to the squeals of laughter and shouts of activity that drift your way on the gentle breeze. . . .

A number of children are at play in the distance, some in groups, some alone. Watch their graceful movements as they chase, swing, slide, build, and climb about the playground. . . .

Moving over to a park bench close by, sit down where you

can see the children easily. Then, when you are ready, as if you are calling to a niece or a nephew you have not seen in many years, call out your name and wait for a reply.

It may take more than a moment, but finally you notice one child respond to your call and begin to make his or her way in your direction. . . . As you watch, without judgment or expectation, notice the dress, bearing, and energy level of your Inner Child as he or she approaches. When close enough, you can see the look of curiosity on his or her face and sense the level of trust in his or her eyes. At a certain distance he or she stops, waiting for the next step to be taken.

You do not need to do or say anything at this time, just observe and note what you see and sense. Action and interaction will come later; for now, simply notice whatever is there for you in this moment of meeting.

This is the child-energy that came into the world with you, the embodiment of curiosity, eagerness, spontaneity, playfulness, wonder, and joy. This is the child that has been with you from the very beginning, helping you, guiding you, and supporting you with limitless energy, boundless creativity, and infinite love as you grew into the world you were given.

Your Inner Child waits patiently, even now, for your invitation, for your return. Give yourself permission to respond to this child in whatever ways you feel most willing and able to do so. Without expectation or judgment, take this moment to greet your Inner Child in the way that feels best to you. There is no need to hurry or to hold back. . . .

When you have taken all the time you need to meet with your Inner Child, thank him or her for coming and let him or her know that you will return later for another visit. Assure him or her that when you return there will be plenty of time for all the things that need to be said and done.

Standing up from the bench, move slowly back to where you

began and then, in whatever way feels right to you, say good-
bye for now.

As the scene fades, be aware of the room around you and the
sounds and sensations of the moment. Take a deep breath or two,
then slowly stretch and open your eyes, feeling relaxed and alert.

Welcome back.

Take a few moments to sit with the experience, whatever
it was, and the feelings, if any, that it evoked. *All* of our
reactions—positive, negative, confused, frustrated, surprised, even empty or numb—can guide us toward learning something important about ourselves. There is no
right or wrong experience in such a situation. Observing
"just what happened" is the beginning of acceptance and
validation of our own inner life.

Guided visualization rarely turns out the way we expect. The key is to pay attention to what *did* happen, not
to worry about what didn't. If you were alone as you did
the visualization, you might want to write down now
some brief notes about the experience. It's as if waking
from a dream: Capture the details soon enough, and they
will be available for your reflection later on.

If you are sharing this experience with another person,
this is a good time to describe what happened as accurately
as you can, even if what occurred was very different from
what you thought would occur.

It is not unusual for people to have no particular reaction or experience at all. Like other skills, imagery takes
some practice, and often people overlook the small things
that do happen because they don't seem to fit their expectations of the situation.

Whatever the results, take a few minutes to reflect on
them now. Consider these questions, which might help
to clarify some of the information available to you from
the exercise.

What did you expect would happen?

What happened?

If you did notice something about a child, where was the child when you first became aware of him or her?

What was he or she doing?

How old would you say the child was?

Could you get a sense of what clothing the child was wearing?

How did the child react to your call?

What were your feelings as you went through the exercise?

What would you say you've learned so far from the exercise?

If you did try the exercise and finished feeling frustrated and confused about the outcome, you might in fact be experiencing some of the feelings that your "historical" child shares. Try above all not to judge negatively what happened; try to accept it for what it is for now. More clarity may come later.

If you are dealing with years of no contact with this part of yourself, things may need to develop more slowly than you would like in order to build the trusting relationship necessary for further unfolding.

For now, it may be sufficient to have made some contact or even to have attempted some contact. Honor your experience whatever it was. When you are ready, you can go further toward establishing communication with the child within.

If you simply did not have a very strong response the first time, you may want to repeat this exercise once or twice more. Just keep track of the things you notice as you go. *Many times, it is the very reaction we dismiss that holds the key to a new understanding of our inner life.*

Consider this a search for a very precious part of yourself and carefully examine any clue at all that presents itself, no matter in what disguise.

When you are ready we can go a step further.

Communicating

Even if you didn't have a clear image of your Inner Child as a result of the visualization above, the next step may still generate some useful information for you. We will be contacting that part of ourselves that is responsible for our childlike energy and initiating communication with it if we can.

Allowing for whatever response we get without negative judgment, let's visit once again the child within. Relax your body, release your breathing, and, gently closing your eyes, recall what you experienced when you made contact with your Inner Child. See yourself once again in the setting where you met with your Inner Child the first time. Establish contact in some way, if you can, with this image of your childlike energy. Be aware of the form and feeling of this valuable part of you. . . .

Sense in whatever way is best for you the specific qualities of your Inner Child as it is now. Acknowledge the courage, endurance, and value this child brings to your life even when you are not aware of it.

Invite your Inner Child to communicate with you more clearly now what you need to know in order to continue to learn and grow.

When you have a sense of contact with your Inner Child, offer to spend some time playing with him or her. Since you are here to learn more about your Inner Child, let yourself be led by your child in whatever way he or she feels most comfortable playing for now.

Since this is still in the realm of the creative imagination, imagine that whatever play environment your child would want to find is available to you now for your play together. Without any expectations about what you must do, spend some time now with your child doing what the two of you wish to do. Try to follow the lead of your child as that feels appropriate. Go anywhere you wish and import anything you would like to play with. Take as much time as you wish to get re-acquainted and to enjoy this time together. . . .

When you have had a chance to "be together" for a while, begin to explore more directly what you can learn from your Inner Child.

Ask your Inner Child specifically what he or she needs from you right now and then wait quietly within for a response. . . . Letting go of your expectations, pay attention to whatever occurs and observe your reaction to it. As if you were listening to a beloved niece or nephew, accept what you hear, feel, or sense without judgment even though you may not understand what it means. . . .

Ask next how your child has been serving you. All of these years, even though out of sight and mind, your Inner Child has been with you, doing its best to protect and care for you. Whatever its "behavior" has been, ask how that has been helpful to you.

When you are ready, ask finally what your Inner Child has to offer you. The response may be surprising or unexpected, but notice it nonetheless.

Recognizing that this is just the beginning of a relationship, let go of any strong expectations you may have about the outcome and offer in return the sort of attention, acceptance, and validation that every child needs and deserves. . . .

When it feels appropriate, send thanks for what you have heard, felt, or sensed and say good-bye for now.

Bringing with you what is most useful to you, slowly become aware of your present surroundings, opening your eyes and stretching easily as you "wake up" feeling rested and refreshed.

As with the first exercise, take some time now to reflect on what occurred as you established communication with your Inner Child. Notice how it felt to play once again with a trusted friend. Consider what you learned and felt in response to the three questions you asked.

It may be that nothing happened in quite the way you wished or expected. That may also have been true in some sense with your own experience as a child. In such cases, it might be tempting to discount or dismiss the value of your efforts. That isn't necessary.

Not everyone processes information in the same way internally. Many people do "see" things easily as if on an internal screen, but others prefer "hearing" or "feeling" as their mode of access. Some people simply find it more difficult than others to interact with their creative imagination. It is a skill they have not exercised much in their lives and, when that is the case, it takes more time and effort to produce results. One strength so valuable in the young, however, is their willingness to persevere until they achieve what they need to. We can all learn from that.

You may have found it possible to contact your Inner Child only to find him or her apparently in great need or even despair. While that can be frightening or feel overwhelming, there is hope in recognizing that "reality."

For whatever reasons, there may have been many unmet needs in your childhood that remain a part of your experience even as an adult. As you reconnect with this "historical" part of the child within you, these feelings and needs may be most prominent for now. Acknowledging them, however, gives you the opportunity then to take action to meet those needs and provide the safety, support, and love that you may have lacked early on.

It could be that you were able to connect with your "child" and found him or her to be an unexpected source of hope, help, and happiness. Do not take that experience for less than its full worth. Contacting the energy and expressiveness of your Inner Child can unlock your creative spirit and inspire in you a greater zest for life.

Whatever experience you had, by becoming aware of the needs as well as the positive energy you felt as a child, you may be better able to make the most of being an adult.

One Person's Journey

After a one-day workshop we did for a group of Adult Children of Alcoholics, we received a letter from one of the participants. It was such an eloquent example of the power of our Inner Child to bring healing that we share parts of it here with you.

It is inspiring evidence that a life filled with pain can still overflow with joy.

"Hello, dear friends! I just wanted to thank you for an absolutely terrific Saturday. I laughed more in that one day I think, than all the rest of my life put together. I cried a lot, too, but I already knew how to do that and these tears were different somehow. All I have to do is think of that day and my heart is filled with love and laughter that reaches from deep inside of me to every part of my being. It puts a sparkle in my eyes and one in my smile that I shall always treasure. . . .

"One of the very special parts to me about Saturday was when you had us lay on the floor and get in touch with the child within. I was surprised because instead of one child inside there were six who were all me and each one looked so different. I tried to do what you said, but there were too many and I felt overwhelmed trying to hold 6 three-year-old children all at the same time (and they didn't seem to want to take turns). So I went back farther in my mind until there was only one. She looked like me when I was very small. She had blonde hair instead of brown and blue eyes instead of dark green.

"I saw me sitting in a crib and then instead of seeing the child, I became the child and at that moment I felt the most incredible sense of wholeness I have ever felt. All my emotions were there in total freedom and purity. I felt the wonder and awe of that completeness and the memory of that has healed me so much.

"I saw morning sunshine filtering through a crack in the curtains and I felt myself reaching for that ray of light that landed on the blanket beside me. I felt my hand reaching for it in wonder and delight trying to grasp it with tiny fingers. I felt the frustration and amazement that I could not catch ahold of it. I felt intense concentration trying to grab the little lint particles that floated in the light. I tried to pick the light up off the blanket, it would get on my hand, but not in it. I felt the contented resignation and acceptance that sunshine wasn't something you hold, but rather something you feel and see.

"I felt my helplessness and dependency on others for my needs as I tried to reach a toy that had fallen on the floor beside the crib. I felt my sadness and impatience waiting for someone to wake up and come get me.

"This memory is very special to me and I share it with you because it taught and gave me so much even though it sounds so simple. All the emotions were there and each one felt good and right. The distortions and ugliness that twisted the beauty in my past were gone and I felt emotional wholeness and goodness as I'm sure God intended them to be.

"The remainder of the day all the children in me were safe and free with all their emotions and secrets of the past and they all blended into me. I met a new me that could laugh and feel joy straight from the heart. No one can ever take that away from me again! That whole day the child in me was touched and loved in safety and peace with joy that seemed to fill and make up for the many years of emptiness and pain and fear. . . . I was wonderfully free at last!

"I thank you both for an incredibly beautiful experience, one so precious to me that words cannot say what is in my heart. May the dear Lord bless you and continue to guide you in your work and lives. Take care and be well.

"Love always,
Sandy"

Thank *you*, Sandy, for all of us.
It *is* never too late.

A Commitment to Caring

What remains is to translate the experience you have had into action you can take to free the child within and find yourself as well. As you develop a dialogue with the playful side of yourself, it is important to validate the messages you are receiving by *acting* on them.

Earlier in the New Game Plan we had you do a *Fun List* (don't you think it is about time you got around to that?). You can now enlist the energy and insight of your own Inner Child to help you expand and refine your list of options and activities and to increase the level of playfulness and pleasure you create in your life.

Check in with your Inner Child to see what would feel good right now. What could you do and who could you do it with if your job was to nourish yourself for the next few minutes, hours, or days? Letting your imagination go where it will, begin to make an expanded fun list that can give you a wealth of choices for celebrating yourself with others.

If it helps, think back to the Guided Replay to connect with the playful experiences you enjoyed as a child. What seems to resonate in you as you recall and read about children at play? How can you translate that energy into something you can do now as an adult? Determine what you are willing to commit to doing now in order to nourish the child within you. If you don't, who will?

By paying attention to the child in yourself and spending some time together in pleasurable ways on a regular basis, you can make a priceless investment in the present moment that will enrich your future. The returns are well worth the risk.

It isn't necessary to force yourself in this process. In fact, making an all-out effort is often just another way to create resistance to change. Barry Stevens, in a book called

Awareness, eloquently describes the results of *struggling* to change.

> When you try to change, you manipulate and torture yourself, and mostly you just become divided between a part of you that tries to change and a part of you that resists change. Even when you do accomplish change in this way, the price is conflict, confusion and uncertainty. Usually, the more you try to change, the worse your situation becomes. . . . It is more useful to simply become aware of yourself as you are now. Rather than try to change, stop, or avoid something that you don't like in yourself, it is much more effective to stay with it and become more deeply aware of it.
>
> When you really get in touch with your own experiencing, you will find that change takes place by itself, without your effort or planning. With full awareness you can let happen whatever wants to happen, with confidence that it will work out well. You can learn to let go and live and flow with your experiencing and happening instead of frustrating yourself with demands to be different. All that energy that is locked up in the battle between trying to change and resisting change can become available for participating in the happening of your life.

Children don't try to "change," they just try something new until they are tired of trying, then they get on with something else until it is time to try again. Their perseverance is always tempered by their desire to feel good about themselves. For children, the ends don't justify the means, rather it is quite the reverse. If the effort is no fun and is damaging to their self-esteem, they find something else to do.

Learn a lesson from your child and value yourself

enough to do something positive and rewarding each day, even if it is something small.

Now as the next step of the New Game Plan for Recovery, we would like you to write a letter to this special child you have just discovered in your life. Put it in your Play Journal and begin it with, perhaps, the salutation "To My Dearest Child."

In this letter we want you to tell the truth about your feelings, hopes, and dreams for your Inner Child. Invite your Inner Child to become a permanent part of your life, bringing with him or her all of the unique positive qualities children so often demonstrate. Finally, tell your child what you are willing to do now to reconnect with this important part of yourself so that you can incorporate its strengths and joys into your adult life.

We have found that the act of committing words to paper, even of an imaginary conversation, serves to make our message that much clearer, our intention that much stronger and our pledge that much more real to us. Just "thinking about it" is not enough to initiate change.

When your letter is finished, read it over again with your Inner Child in mind. Then, in your creative imagination, make contact once again with your Inner Child and take him or her onto your lap and into your arms. In whatever way feels right to you, share your letter with him or her.

Clearly express to him or her what you are willing to do to create a stronger relationship.

Share your readiness to allow a new level of spontaneity, delight, and adventure into your daily activities.

. Indicate your openness to inviting a sense of wonder and awe, curiosity and creativity into your interactions with others.

Communicate your commitment to care for, support, and

nourish the child within you as if it were as precious as any other child in the world.

For you, it is!

When you are ready, return to the "real" world with a renewed sense of acceptance, excitement, and hope for the new day dawning in your life.

It *is* possible to be free.

4

A Sense of Play

*A person will be called
to account on Judgment Day
for every permissible thing
he might have enjoyed—
but did not.*
THE TALMUD

Permission to play: There's the rub.

When we ask people to write about what keeps them from playing more in their lives, the responses we get are often very similar. People write about too much stress, job pressures, too little time, not enough energy, and the like. Then there are the themes of fear, judgment, embarrassment, rejection . . . and finally we also see the notion that play is not serious business, not worthwhile or productive. Some sample responses by our workshop participants suggest the tone these comments often convey:

The major blocks to playing that I am aware of are:

Too tired to play after work. STRESS! I have to be serious.

Embarrassment, being uncomfortable with others, fear of not being accepted.

I feel silly. I feel too big. (I've always been very tall and never felt like a kid.) Someone might look at me and see I'm not perfect. I usually don't like or want to play. This makes me feel sad for myself.

The shame I learned from childhood that playing is noisy, unproductive, and bothersome to adults. To play is to be careless and unproductive.

Fear of opinion of others. Belief that it is a waste of time—of no value. Can't think of anything fun to do.

And in answering the question of how they feel when they play, the responses are reflections of guilt, tension, and irresponsibility almost as much as they are of delight, joy, freedom, and energy. For example:

When I play I feel:

Silly. Like I should remember I'm a grown-up. That play is for others. I should apologize or feel guilty if I play.

Like it has to be fast and furious because it will go away and I'll have to be serious again.

Guilty for having such a good time and I usually seek to punish myself in some fashion, i.e., self-incrimination.

Guilty—disapproval—uptight.

When we ask how people play now in their life, the most common answer of all is with kids—sons, daughters, a friend's children, and so forth. Pets come into the picture, too, like the one belonging to the woman who wrote that her way of playing is "running screaming through the house with my Doberman until she knocks me down."

But all too often the response is left blank or simply filled with such words as, "I don't, unless something like this encourages me."

It isn't all that bad, of course. Many more positive responses are included along the way. But the clear indication is that as adults we have a terribly difficult time justifying, generating, and enjoying pure play. It usually gets second or third priority at best. We are an affluent society, yet it seems that we have less leisure time than ever before and that the use we make of it is less rewarding than it might be.

For some people the material we have already presented is more than enough to remind them of the power of play in their lives. With a sigh of recognition and a surge of energy they continue the journey they never really left. For them the experience is one of validation more than anything else. They are already on the path.

For others the process is one of gaining permission for their creative, imaginative, expressive side to emerge. They have remained in touch with those skills, but have felt some inhibition and constraint about revealing them very openly to others. They may have a rich inner life and a developed sense of humor, but they have held it back from the world in order to protect it or themselves from the risk of exposure.

Once convinced of a safe enough environment, they often surprise their friends and family with the depth and richness of those inner resources. Realizing *where* the permission needs to come from is usually the biggest step in such cases.

Then there are the people who have no real idea what we are talking about when we speak of play, delight, joy, or the Inner Child. They know they must have been a child once; but they know that only in an intellectual way, not from their recollection of it. For many reasons, their experience of their childhood and the powers that came with it are hidden from them behind a thick wall or a heavy fog.

For these people validation and permission are not enough. They need acceptance, understanding, guidance, *and* patience. They need time and space in which to begin again, as if for the first time. These are gifts that they must give themselves.

In order to be of service to any and all of these people, we will spend some time now exploring the process of play through some specific sets of activities and exercises. They are designed to encourage the reader's involvement, exploration, and initiative in creating playful experiences and interactions.

If these exercises serve to stimulate or suggest other playful activities that may feel more appropriate and rewarding, then they have achieved their purpose. Feel free to improvise and improve upon them.

In this chapter and the next one we focus on readers' own creation of personally satisfying play experiences. Chapter 6 will expand that focus to include close relationships and the family and will outline some of the boundaries of play, suggesting guidelines for avoiding misuse or abuse of play. In chapter 7 we will look at ways to bring play even into the world of work.

Our goal will be to help those who need some of that validation, permission, acceptance, encouragement, and guidance in order to finally find their way back to the playful energy within them.

Guidelines to Good Times

Where do we begin?

With ourselves. We need to move once more back into our bodies and energize our senses. It is there that we began and there we can find renewal. We need to get in contact again with Nature, with the rhythms and cycles of our birthplace in the universe. We need to activate our intellect and exercise our emotions, to stay alert to and expressive of the wonders and delights that surround us. With all that in mind, the next series of exercises focuses on pleasurable activities, pastimes, and assignments.

We'll also give you some guidelines designed to increase your chances for success in this new endeavor. Be absolutely sure to follow them exactly as much as you feel like.

Guideline #1: Start small.

Think for a minute what kind and level of expectations we have for three-week-old children. If they look at us for more than a minute at a time or smile briefly in our direction, we are delighted. Even if others call it gas, we know inside they *are* making contact with us. We are as happy when they are asleep as when they are awake. Often we're happier.

It can be the same way for us as we learn once more

how to play. If we can just set our sights on creating five minutes of pleasure each day, we may find ourselves much more likely to follow through than if our expectations consistently exceed our abilities. We don't have to become experts immediately, that is too much like what happens when we "grow up." Nourish the infant child within and let the growing take care of itself.

Guideline #2: Don't force it.

When your *idea* of play takes the place of playing, the life goes out of the experience. That is not to say you should not play with ideas—some of our finest philosophy, poetry, and drama come from such pastimes—but it is important not to lose the *feeling* of play as you toy with whatever medium is at hand. When the spark is gone or the fantasy vanishes, let go of the effort and move on to something else. You have nothing to prove by pushing.

You will also find that pressure never seems to work when you attempt to get others to play with you. Remember that play is a voluntary practice, and one that often takes as long to create as it does to experience. Make the negotiations with others a part of the play by using your imagination to come up with several options—some of them, at least, outlandish. Then be sure to select something that all present can be happy with. Enthusiastic playmates make the process more fun, and everyone benefits.

Guideline #3: Let your play define itself.

Many times the difficulty comes from our playing not like we *want* to play but, rather, like we *ought* to play. We may compare ourselves to others and imitate their actions. In short, we play by other people's rules, and in that bargain we discount the small sparks of joy struck by our activity. That discounting insures that we will experience fewer and fewer of those sparks.

Play is an attitude and an experience, not a form or a formula. It is not so much *what* we do as it is *how* we do it. Only *you* know what feels good to you. Honor that feeling.

Guideline #4: Create space for your explorations.

Play can get crowded out by all of the other "important" things in life, if you let it. Or it can be an integral part of everything you do. If you allow your playful, wondering, curious child to accompany you—that child you've already made contact with—you can begin to have fun with whatever is before you at the moment.

Begin reserving those few minutes of enjoyment a few times a day, no matter where you are. Whether the setting is your rustling up breakfast in the morning, driving to the office, working on the job, or spending Sunday afternoon with the family, you can find ways to play.

Making a commitment is important. The value we give to playing is only as great as our willingness to make it a priority in our lives. But that does not mean that we now have yet another opportunity to criticize, judge, or blame ourselves if we don't play exactly as we planned. *Allowing* a playful attitude and joyful experience into our daily routine is more valuable than forcing one. As we shall see in chapter five, force and play do not coexist.

Recognize any feeling of guilt for what it often is, a reflection of messages we received as children. Refuse to support those messages any longer: Set aside that time to play at regular intervals *and* play regularly whether you have set aside the time or not. Your Inner Child will notice the change.

Guideline #5: Reward yourself.

Value your play enough to invest in the things that bring you pleasure. Collect your own set of "toys" to play with.

Find those places you have always wanted to go to but have never quite gotten to.

Begin now by deciding to create some real "play money." How much are you willing to set aside from your weekly pay to devote purely to play? The amount is not critical, make it something you can truly afford. Get yourself a piggy bank to hold your weekly allotment and be sure you spend it *all* up each week—no carryovers!

This is not a limited account. You may make additional deposits at will; the only restriction is that you not let it lie untouched for more than a week. If you accidentally forget to spend it *all* one week, you must put in *double* that amount *extra* the next week! That is our way of assuring your increasing "interest" in play.

It may be only a few bucks a week; but each time you buy yourself something just because it is fun to play with or go someplace because it makes you feel good, you are validating your right to enjoy life and creating another connection to your Inner Child. And make sure your toys are really *your* toys—remember Guideline 3!

Perhaps your playhouse is a bookstore rather than a toy shop; or it's a stationery store, or a hardware outlet. Wherever you feel a sense of delight and excitement, give yourself permission to fully explore and enjoy the experience. Pick out a place you have been longing to "mess around" in and go mess. Just be sure to clean up before you leave.

You are a source of your own pleasure. As you invest yourself you will receive the rewards. No one can play for you, and no one else can reward you without your involvement and acceptance of the gift. Value yourself and your Inner Child enough to invite wonder, curiosity, and fun back into your life each day.

Since we ourselves can't remember much more than five things at once, we will leave it there for now. Whether you try out some of the things we suggest or ditch this book and get on with playing, just keep those guidelines in mind and you will do great. Your Inner Child knows what to do anyway, you merely need to learn how to listen.

Making Sense of It All

Let us now focus our attention on ways to engage in play through the magic of our senses. That is where we all started, learning about the world through our skin and muscles, sensation and movement. (In chapter 5 we will move in the other direction, inwardly, since there is more than just one world in which to play.)

For a more in-depth treatment of this topic we heartily recommend *Healthy Pleasures*, a book by Robert Ornstein and David Sobel. It is one of the most thorough, balanced, and practical books we have seen on how to feel good and enjoy life. It is well worth searching for (and acting on)! With any luck you can do as we have and steal some great ideas on how to have fun.

The activities that follow are all exploratory in nature. The order is somewhat arbitrary. They are intended to be a framework rather than a straightjacket. Since this is a book for adults, you may make them downright sensual if you would like.

The thing to keep in mind is that *the means must justify the ends*. Take a risk or two in trying them out, be prepared for some uncomfortable moments as you engage in new behavior, but trust your sense of yourself to tell you which ones work and which ones don't.

Let go, with no guilt, of the ones that don't. Play around with the ones that do. If you come up with some interesting variations, let us know. Who can tell what we might include in our second book, *The New Game Plan, Too*.

Touch:

We will begin, like Ornstein and Sobel, with the sense of touch. It is surely one of the most basic of the senses and one of the most neglected in our modern society and culture.

The amount of skin-to-skin contact between a mother and a newborn is essential for the development of the entire nervous system, with certain levels of brain growth being affected as much as fifteen years later. Psychologists have found that deprivation of nurturing touch can lead to death in severely neglected infants.

While we may not be able to go back and address those issues at this time in our life, we can at least recognize the power of the sense of touch and insure that from now on we don't continue any lack of such contact with the world. From the more positive viewpoint, the payoff for enhancing our experience can be profoundly rewarding.

Go over your Fun List (see, we told you to get it done!) and identify any of the things you already know you enjoy that have a strong element of touch associated with them. Then waste no time in getting to them. (Short on

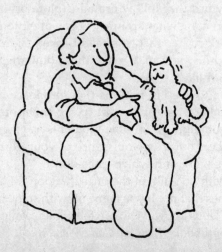

cash? Try "trading" massages with a friend or lover instead of paying an outsider for them. The rewards are physical as well as financial—an excellent example of giving and receiving becoming one!)

See if you can come up with five *more* fun things that you used to do or want to do that qualify in this category and add them to your overall list. But don't stop there, be sure to try some of them out.

If you are running out of possibilities, then we suggest you invest a couple of bucks in a marvelously plastic and malleable substance that we all have played with at some time as kids, namely, the earth. Good quality clay is about as natural and enduring a medium as humankind has ever known. It is inexpensive, readily available in most cities, towns, or riverbeds, and suitable for people of all levels of skill and experience.

It has limitless potential for imaginative and creative interaction on sensory, aesthetic, expressive, and even functional levels. There is no right or wrong way to play with it (unless you mind cleaning up messes), and it is completely recyclable within the privacy of your own home. (That means you can squash up anything you don't want anyone else to see and then have another go at it later on.)

Get some. Clear a large space at the kitchen table or on the back porch. Put on some old clothes and take off your watch and ring. Get your hands wet and go at it.

Take your time to savor the sensations. Notice the associations that come up as you play with the clay. Invite your Inner Child to join you and even to become your guide.

Remember the mud pies and the mud puddles, the play dough and the modeling clay? Remember the hours of molding and mashing, pounding and pressing that filled your days at some time in your life? Remember the digging and planting, the kneading and rolling, the squeezing and stretching that absorbed your attention until you were lost in them? And if you *can't* remember, *then by all means experience them now.*

Don't "make" anything. Just mess around. Go slow. Try out different amounts of water, different amounts of clay. Use your elbow, your knuckles, your fingernails, your knees. See how thin you can make it, how round, how tall, how intricate. Cut it, weave it, throw it, shape it. Listen with your body and speak with your hands. Stay with the process as long as you can.

Close your eyes and listen. Silence your mind and look. Savor the deep, rich scent of our Mother Earth. Tease out the textures of the everchanging clay. Give yourself a chance to become one with your ancient ancestors as they sat by the riverbed fashioning their implements of survival and ceremony, molding meaning out of matter in the morning sun.

Challenge yourself to do something specific only if you must and *after* you have fully explored the medium. Then try not to judge the results immediately. And when you are done, be sure to enjoy washing up afterward as much as you enjoyed messing up initially.

Carry that same level of attentiveness into the other parts of your world and you will find it possible to find pleasure anywhere.

Doing it can be even more fun than thinking about it.

Taste:

Our palates have been dulled by fast food flavorings and monotonous meals. We have been freeze dried, frozen, packaged, and processed until convenience takes precedence over taste and texture. Consistency is valued more than variation and predictability has priority above spontaneity. In the press of the day we give up taste in favor of function and often see our meals as interruptions to be tolerated rather than celebrated.

It is time to change.

We can begin by setting aside special times to honor our eating and begin doing it in a new way. It may be enjoyable to join with others for an evening out, but it can also be interesting to take our Inner Child out for a meal by ourselves so that we can concentrate on the experience more than on interaction with others.

Think about the places you typically frequent for food—even if "frequent" doesn't quite apply because you seldom eat out. Often we have developed a taste for a certain cuisine or a favorite type of meal. An alternative to noting the places you most enjoy is to pay attention to the types of food you have specifically *not* tried out yet. Exploring something new can be fun if you allow for unexpected sensations along the way.

Use the phone book or a local tourist brochure to locate a restaurant that serves a type of food you have little or no experience with. Give yourself permission to try it out without too many preplanned responses. Be bold. Explore the exotic. Try out something you would not normally choose. Pay attention to the taste, the texture, the scents. Allow yourself to be pleased or not, depending on the experience, not on the expectation. See if you can expand your range of options and your limits of "like-ability."

Don't hold back. Order that appetizer, eat that dessert! Pretend you are the food critic for your local newspaper or a national travel guide and consider how many stars you would give to the experience. Move upscale or get down home and have a ball.

You could even pretend to be a tourist from Toronto on vacation and quiz the waitpeople about the curious customs of the locals. The trick is to get out of your ordinary routine enough to taste life from a new perspective. If you don't know how, ask for help—your Inner Child is great at pretending.

Write up that review in your journal or diary. Make the recommendations and draw in the stars. Share your results with someone you know and get a recommendation from him or her for another restaurant or food to try. Experiment. Expect the unexpected. Accept the results with a smile.

Of course you have probably realized by now there is an even better way to experience the expansion of your sense of taste—cook that food yourself! This option has the added advantage of combining sensations from several senses at once.

The sense of touch as you select, sort, wash, chop, and serve the food; the sense of smell as you fill the kitchen with the aromas of the cooking meal; the sense of sound as the boiling, broiling, frying, steaming and spilling take place; the sense of sight as you observe the myriad of changes that occur as you prepare, dish up, and serve the meal; and the sense of taste we started to focus on in the beginning as you snitch, test, clean up, and ultimately finish off the food.

Many forms of cooking can be particularly wonderful blends involving all our senses—baking bread, for example, or preparing a multicolored fruit salad (with nothing out of a can!). A spicy Indian curry or old-fashioned stew can add excitement to the last of the leftover vegetables, and a traditional potluck dinner is fun for everyone (and usually provides several new—and sometimes intimidating—offerings).

When you try out something new and unusual, even if it turns out terrible, you will have the fun of describing it to others (once your stomach settles down and the oven finally gets cleaned out).

Those of you with particularly trustworthy friends might try out an exciting taste experience by becoming a taster! Now, of course, you know that tasters have to be impartial and unbiased. As a result they often engage in "blind" taste testing so that they will be able to remain neutral as they assess the experience.

Your job is to find people creative enough to come up with several taste sensations and who will give them to you while *you* are blindfolded. If they have kept their treats a secret and keep you guessing what's coming next, you will learn some exciting new things about the value and function of your sense of taste. Just make sure your friends agree to switching roles at some point—that should insure that they remain compassionate as they choose their menu.

If you are truly research-minded and wish to engage in double-blind testing, remember to spread plenty of towels or newspapers around first so you and your blindfolded friend won't have to worry too much about the mess that will be created in the interests of scientific progress.

Playing with the transformative energy of fire through cooking can be as rewarding as interacting with the slow, solid substance of the earth. Both have been with us from

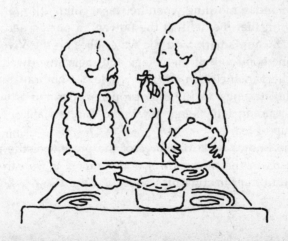

the beginning and offer endless opportunities for further exploration and play.

Remember, it is *how* you invest your energy and attention that makes the pleasure possible. It *is* possible to find a way to have more fun even when doing what you have to do. It just takes some imagination, innovation, creativity, and, often, the participation of someone you enjoy being with.

You can also have some fun even on your own as you follow your sense of taste back into your past experiences of pleasure. Sometimes our body-sense allows us to access memories that are unavailable to our more rational recollections.

The potential impact of such recollections is perhaps nowhere more powerfully illustrated than in that monumental work of Marcel Proust's, *Remembrance of Things Past*.

In this classic collection of writings, Proust describes with incredible clarity how the world of his youth—houses, gardens, streets, and more—came back to him as an adult when he recognized the taste of a small breakfast cake dipped in tea, the treat his aunt used to give to him on a Sunday morning when he was a child.

"So in that moment all the flowers in our garden and in M. Swann's park, and the water-lilies on the Vivonne and the good folk of the village and their little dwellings and the parish church and the whole of Combray and of its surroundings, taking their proper shapes and growing solid, sprang into being, town and gardens alike, from my cup of tea."

Who knows what treasures of the present or the past await us in the next morsel or fragrance, if we can but attend to their fleeting message.

Smell:

This one fits well along with the category above, since taste is nonexistent without the sense of smell.

In addition to the ideas suggested above, you might spend some time recollecting the special scents and smells of your childhood, especially the ones that you associate with pleasurable experiences. Perhaps it is the buttery smell of fresh popcorn in the darkness of a movie theater, or the cinnamony scent of apple cider at Halloween. Maybe it is the fresh-green fragrance of a bright spring morning, or the crisp, acrid odor of burning leaves on a fall afternoon. Or, unawares, you suddenly catch the scent of a certain cologne and vividly recall your very first date, so many years ago.

The air can hold a treasure of memories if we allow ourselves to resonate with them. Whenever your sense of

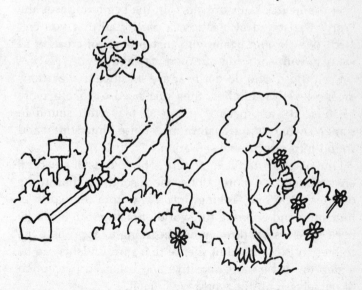

smell uplifts your spirits, pay attention to the experience. It may be one you can come back to later on to explore more fully. The gift you discover as a result may be one given to you first when you were a child.

Hearing:

We are a culture that is bound by sound. Silence is the one thing we rarely hear. The problem with the glut of noise, the traffic, the sirens, the airplanes, the air conditioners, the radios, the stereos, the telephones, the televisions, is that they are too much with us. We very rarely pay conscious attention to them.

We have learned by necessity to tune them out, to turn them off, effectively, though they "play" on. Our sensitivity to sound has been deadened, our appreciation dulled. We are lost in sound and lost without it.

We must reclaim the power of sound, of vibration, that is at the heart of our universe. In the beginning was the Word, the sound of creation, a part of all that was created. We can join again with that process of creation as we play with sound in our own way and day.

Even those who do not hear are sensitive to vibrations of one level or another, they just need to take a more "hands on" approach. We can all play with sound in some way or other, transforming "noise" into sound and sound into pleasurable sensation.

One place to start is in Nature. The sounds of a natural environment are more subtle, more soothing than those of a technical one. Taking time away from the world of humanity and entering the world of Nature can begin by itself to refresh and renew us. Learning to appreciate the fullness of sound and of silence that surrounds us can be a step toward a more sensitive and balanced perception of ourselves and the world we inhabit.

Another way to play is by creating sounds, by setting

the very air to sing. This is another basic, traditional form of play. It is a form of communication, but rarely utilitarian in nature. It is at the heart of all rituals. It can be a process of attunement and a practice of self-expression. It can be an act of renewal and celebration. It is interesting to note that no one "works" a sound-producing instrument.

If you have ever before trained on some musical instrument, you may have to overcome the negative impact of that experience; but the attempt is worth the effort. The trick is to "unlearn" enough to get back to the creative, playful stage of simply interacting with sound and appreciating the results no matter how curious or unexpected they may be.

If you have never studied music or been a musician, so much the better. You can start with "beginner's mind" and allow your Inner Child to lead the way. We recommend that you pick an instrument that is not technically demanding in the early stages of learning. A drum, a piano, a guitar, a penny whistle can all be suitable selections. Glass jars filled with varying amounts of water, kazoos, slide whistles, or wind chimes can also fill the bill.

Whatever it is, the task is to explore it, to stretch its possibilities, to toy with the range of sound you can create with it, to enter into it and join with it as it resonates with the universe.

As with the clay and the fire we spoke of earlier, it is the interaction with the medium that is important, not the outcome. Not all sounds are pleasant, nor should they be. Sounds can be attractive or repulsive—as any competent four-year-old will immediately demonstrate! We are not suggesting you make music so much as that you play with sounds. Of course, for those who already enjoy making music we will not deny them the experience, just suggest they may want to "play" a little first.

Let's say you found a drum. The ones made by native artisans out of traditional materials offer some of the most rewarding of responses, but any drum or turned-over trash can will do. Look at it carefully, note the colors, the materials, the construction. Pick it up. Feel the weight, the substance of it. Notice where it is hard, where it gives to pressure, where it moves.

Using your hands, your fingers, tap on it, thump it, slap it softly. Pay attention to the variation in sounds that come from different parts of the drum, different locations on it. Vary the strength of the strike, try out various implements to strike with. If there is an open end, cover and uncover it. Hold it between your knees, place it on the ground, set it on a chair. In a variety of ways see how many sounds you can coax from this instrument and listen to the particular message each sound conveys.

Tune the drum by adding tension or pressure to the surface as you play. Try sliding your fingers across the top, gently scratching the skin, dropping small objects onto the surface to find out how they respond. In whatever way you can think of (without causing damage) make contact with and interact with this piece of the world.

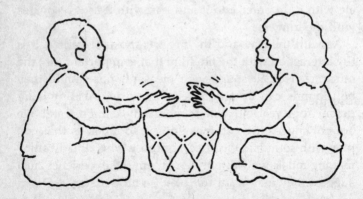

When you have a good sense of the sounds you can make, pay attention to the rhythms that are possible. Play with the speed, the variations, the patterns that occur to you. Find the rhythm of your own heartbeat and the pulse of your own time.

Become the forest dweller calling for success on the hunt, the shaman casting out illness, the plains dweller celebrating the rain, the soldier marching into battle, the percussionist in the symphony orchestra. Let yourself wander through history and around the world, becoming one with the drummers of all time.

For a marvelous journey of this sort, we highly recommend the books and tapes by Mickey Hart, *Drumming at the Edge of Magic* and *Planet Drum*. They are the result of a master at play.

This sort of play is possible, of course, with stringed instruments, flutes, whistles, homemade instruments, whatever is available at the moment. The process is what counts, the result is secondary at this stage. Have fun with it. Mastery can come later as it pleases.

Sight:

Perhaps our most dominant sense of all is sight. It is said that as much as 80 percent of our energy each day is involved in the act of seeing. We are confronted with endless visual stimulation from the moment of waking to the last seconds of activity. Some researchers estimate that television alone contributes an average of seven hours a day of imagery to our modern households. Add in newspapers, magazines, billboards, and product packaging, and we are awash in a sea of visual sensations.

To transform the commonplace into the uniquely satisfying is no easy trick. To play with our visual sense we must find a way to activate our imagination, to interact with images in a new way. Artists are in the business of such play, but we can all take part in the process whether anyone else sees the outcome or not.

We suggest that you consider color as a primary access point, the more free-flowing the better. Finger paints are a favorite of the kindergarten set for good reason: The act of merging color and form through touch and movement is extremely satisfying. The ''hows'' and ''whys'' disappear as the involvement increases and the discoveries take place. Spontaneity and experimentation are almost an obligation as boundaries blur and colors melt together. Even mistakes are just an invitation to another avenue of exploration. This is a world where the Inner Child can truly be our guide.

We recommend using the best quality fingerpaints and paper that you can find. Even they are generally inexpensive, and the better the quality of color you create, the more rewarding the process becomes.

This is one play activity in which you may want to invite a youngster or two to join you. They are an acceptable ''cover'' in case another adult shows up, and they will constantly expand your sense of possibilities—''Oh no! Not the brown and the green. . . . ''

Oil pastels are another favorite of ours. They have intensity of color without the chalky quality of regular pastels. Just making marks on a page can be an intriguing process with this medium. Again, don't try to draw anything, just play with the colors and shapes. See which combinations are the most pleasing, which the least. Get a feel for the energy of certain blends, the emotions that are implied, the textures that you can create.

Make a spontaneous squiggle on the page, then see how many different images it suggests. Turn it on all sides, consider different perspectives, notice what isn't there that could be. If you are playing with a partner, take turns with your marks on the same page without telling the other what you have in mind. Be prepared to find and let go of several images in the process of completing ''one'' picture.

Watercolors are another medium with great possibilities. You can almost guarantee that the hue you intend is not what you will get, so "messing around" becomes almost mandatory. Remember to leave the judgmental side of your nature in the other room as you play. Let the colors flow, then allow the images to emerge. The picture can take on a life of its own at times, turning in a moment from what you had in mind to something entirely different. See if you can follow the changes as they occur.

Then there are kaleidoscopes, cameras, art galleries, and museums, seashores, sunsets, flower gardens and nature trails, city lights, mountain heights, and any number of other ways to experiment with and expand your sense of sight.

Imagine yourself immersed in a world of visual delights.

Since we have covered something from the earth, air, and fire categories, the element of water comes to mind as another medium of play. The sensory pleasure available in a simple tub of hot, bubbly water (perhaps graced by an aromatic oil or two), is legendary. The conviviality that comes from sharing that hot tub with friends is a treat that has been known down the ages.

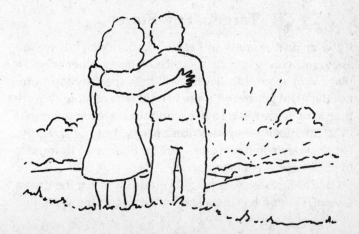

Then there are the more active forms of play involving others as well. How about a good old-fashioned water balloon fight? Or if you are really into intensity, how about a battle to the death with squirt guns? Being confirmed pacifists, we carefully keep all the water pistols for adult use only, we wouldn't want children to get the wrong idea (or the drop on us)!

If you can get to a suitable lake, pond, or river, you can also engage in a form of meditation that is the perfect marriage of earth, air, water, and fire. I am speaking of the ancient art of stone skipping.

By selecting exactly the right sort of stone, choosing the most suitable expanse of water, and allowing precisely for the effect of the wind, you can fire that stone in such a way that it dances delicately across the surface like a drop of water on a hot griddle. There are few thrills to match the perfect throw. And always, there's an even more perfect one waiting in the next stone . . . or the next.

Earth, air, fire, and water, touch, taste, smell, hearing, sight—we hope by now that you are getting the message. And yet this is only the beginning.

Target: Toy Stores

As your next exercise in becoming more playful, we are assigning you a visit to a source of many other ways to play, a toy store. Ideally this will be a specialty toy store, not the giant get-everything-cheaper type of store. We are preparing to gather resources, and what we are interested in is the quality and selection of toys, not the quantity. Go on a day when you can spare an hour or so to wander to your heart's content.

On this first visit (did we tell you this was just the first of several?) your job is to look at everything in the store. Just look (and touch). Pay attention to when your interest is piqued and your curiosity is aroused. Pick things up and toy with them. Allow the memories to come as you stumble across old favorites. Recall, if you can, the different ages and stages when each type of toy might have been most attractive to you. Find out which ones still are. Don't hurry, this is important work. You'll know it's work because we instruct you to leave without buying anything.

On your second visit, pick another store. This time your objective is to select three toys for your Inner Child. This means, of course, that you have to develop a sense of what you might enjoy playing with, too, since the two of you are rather inseparable. Again, look everything over completely before you commit yourself. You can usually tell you are in the right territory when you feel an involuntary smile cross your face as you spot something.

On your third visit your task is to buy a "care" package

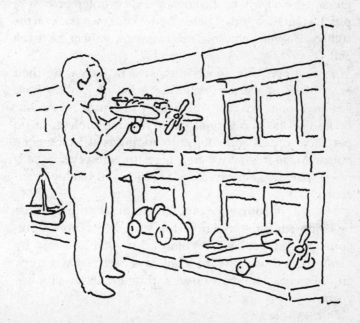

(as in "I care for you") for your closest adult friend. Since you may not know just what he or she would most enjoy, pick out things *you* would enjoy and then at least someone will be sure to be delighted with the gift.

Generally it is wise not to spend too much money; some of the best toys are quite inexpensive and your goal is not to generate a sense of obligation on the part of your friend. And don't forget to *send* the package—you can always get yourself the same things so that the two of you can play together.

The fourth through the hundredth visits are for you alone. It is permissible to buy toys for others as the thought or need arises, but you should always strive to keep your eye out for a new nifty-gifty for yourself. After all, there is that accumulation of "play money" that you have to turn over each week!

Beyond the hundredth visit you will need no further guidance. You will be a certifiable expert in the process of play by that time and eligible to write your own book on the subject. Heaven knows we need as many of them as we can get.

As a support for those interested in increasing their level of play, we are including a list of *toys we know and love*—ones we often play with in groups or on our own. The list is personal, arbitrary, incomplete, in no particular order, and subject to additions at a moment's notice. Most of what we are suggesting, however, is fairly inexpensive, easy to carry around, and readily available.

You are, of course, encouraged to make your own list by completing the assigned toy store visits, consulting your Guided Replay for "oldies but goodies," and by hauling out those gifts from holidays past that you stuck on the shelf of the hall closet and forgot about all these years.

Our favorites:

Active Toys:

soft fabric "flippy flyers"—like Frisbees, only they fold up and fit in your pocket and can be thrown indoors without breaking *too* many things.

Frisbees—in a variety of shapes, sizes, materials, and styles. Foam, rubber, or paper ones can be used indoors. Disc golf is a great game you can play anywhere outdoors (in addition to plain old catch), and you can design the course as you go along. Aerobies are amazing, the jet set of discs.

juggling balls—soft ones, bouncy ones, ones with funny shapes. Juggling can be learned with perseverance and a little time, and there is no end to the level of challenge available. A great stress-reducer (once you've learned how to juggle!) and not bad for reducing other things if you have to pick up your mistakes very often. Hints: Get *Juggling for the Complete Klutz* and juggle standing next to your bed, you don't have to bend so far to "collect yourself." Also, very sheer scarves are an easy (slow-speed) way to begin.

hackey sack—not everyone's cup of tea, but fun once you get the hang of it. This is a small leather bag that you keep in play by kicking with the side of your foot. You *can* learn, honest! If you can't, get three of them and juggle 'em!

Koosh balls—a weird, wiggly rubber-band sort of ball that just feels good to fiddle with. Good for juggling, petting, spinning by one strand, talking to . . .

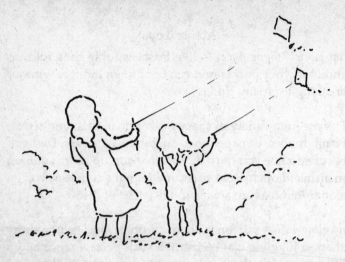

flying things—paper airplanes, balsa wood airplanes, kites (regular, stunt, fighter, exotic, etc.), water-filled rockets (for shooting at airplanes), parachutes (for launching from high-flying kite after airplane has been hit by a rocket).

bubbles—great for picnics, parties, and pacifying rowdy kids. Bubbles from small to gigantic can be blown, most of which have a magical, mysterious resemblance to a certain blue-green planet that circles a small sun in the Milky Way galaxy.

generic sports equipment—all of the regular things we grown-ups think of when we think of play. How we use them is the key to whether they have "play value" or are just another excuse to "work out." When that No. 2 wood sends us into overdrive, we are probably no longer "playing" golf. It *is* possible to finish a game feeling refreshed and renewed no matter what the score would suggest.

Puzzles and Games:

tangrams—originally from China, this fascinating puzzle has over 1,600 design variations possible, and can be played by one or more players. Endlessly challenging.

board games—a variety of ancient and modern games encourage social interaction and enjoyment (and keep you from getting bored). Try some of the traditional ones—mancala, go, backgammon, fox and geese—as well as the contemporary ilk.

card games—from solitaire to bridge, blackjack to hearts, games for every taste, talent, and temperament. It is *not* necessary to bet money in order to have fun. Matchsticks, poker chips, and paper clips can do just fine and are cheaper to give away.

paper and pencil games—crossword puzzles, battleship, hangman, brain-teasers, creativity quizzes, etc. These have the benefit of being highly portable, cheap, and simple enough (*some* of them, anyway) to play with young ones when appropriate.

magic tricks—some very fascinating ones can be purchased at specialty shops for very little money. Once you know how they work, there is still the challenge of pulling off the sleight-of-hand in front of an audience!

puzzles—wooden ones, plastic ones, water-filled ones, impossible ones. Arts and crafts shows often have some beautiful examples of puzzles that are as lovely to look at as they are difficult to solve.

Office and Desk Toys:

Silly Putty—accept no substitutes, the real thing is the one. Great for filling in time while stuck on the phone. Now available in fluorescent colors, too!

finger tops—save at least one empty spot on the desk for a spin while on hold, waiting for a call, brainstorming, etc. There are some elegant ones available in exotic woods. The flat, reflective disks put on quite a show and seem to go on forever.

decorative playthings—sandscapes (sand and colored water framed between two layers of glass), color boxes, liquid timers, whatever you can find that looks attractive and changes every time you give it a flip or a twist. Give the sandscape a spin just as you leave work and see how it turns out the next morning.

trash can "basketball hoops"—some come with their own backboards, some just stick to the wall (for a while). Put the hoop far enough away for a challenge but close enough that you don't get exhausted chasing down your errant missiles (or get embarrassed when someone walks in on the evidence of your ineptitude).

executive desk toys—this usually designates miniature versions of larger games on sale at gigantic prices. It *is* possible to find a gem here or there for less than a fortune, however. The small electronic "blasters" with four to eight deadly weapons plus flashing lights look intriguing (for *after* the boss leaves the room).

flexible sculptures—several varieties; Tangle, a unique, soothing, plastic loop, wraps around itself in a never-ending cycle, reflecting, perhaps, the knots we tie ourselves in regularly. This one doesn't ever unravel completely, but then, we hope, neither do we! There are also geometric figures made of metal that twist and turn into new designs and configurations, a variety of interesting toys that use pendulums, that balance, spin, and turn with fascinating results.

There is, of course, an overwhelming range of playthings that we have not even touched on. Our object is not to be comprehensive, rather it is to be suggestive. The items are less important than the enjoyment they bring. Anything goes. If it delights you it qualifies as a toy. Find your own favorite toys and share them with others in play.

We have even made up for ourselves a backpack of portable playthings that can be grabbed on the way out the door whenever there is the possibility that time to snatch some fun might be found in the near future. Just looking at the bag is enough to recall the powerful, positive benefits of play—that are always within reach, with or without a bag to contain them.

Finally, having made this list of some of our favorite toys, we got so excited that we started a company to provide toys to others who don't have the time or inclination to wander all over town looking for them. Since many of the things we enjoy most are hard to find, we created Playmakers as a direct mail source of toys, publications, and guidance in the world of play.

After years of dedicated research, intensive field testing, and extensive evaluation, we are finally offering to the public by catalog what we would most like to find in our ideal toy store. In fact, we even have plans for a quarterly newsletter and a Toy-of-the-Month Club to provide low-cost, high-quality toys to subscribers the whole year 'round. Truly a gift that keeps on giving! For further information and a catalog, write to us at Playmakers, P. O. Box 90488, Austin, TX 78709 or call us at (512) 346–7529 (PLAY).

There are an infinite number of ways to play with the world. And an infinite number of worlds to play with, as we shall see in the next chapter.

ENJOY!

5

The Journey Inward

*In our innermost soul we are children
and remain so for the rest of our lives.*
FREUD

One thing that unites children and mystics is that they both see the world with luminous, limitless vision. For both, the line between reality and the dream world is not finely drawn or distinct and there exist worlds within worlds. While we may not aspire to mystical perspectives, we can certainly honor the imaginative ones that are our heritage and birthright.

For each of the worldly senses—and some cultures recognize far more of them than others—there are corresponding imaginative ones. We can imagine what someone or something looks like, for example, as well as actually seeing them.

It may well be this quality, which usually reaches its

heights of power in young children, that sets us apart from any other species we know of.

We have access to a special world of memory, expectation, fantasy, and magic, a world curiously free of the constraints of time, space, and resources that operate in the outer environment. By the grace of our imaginative senses, we can appreciate levels of symbol and significance, metaphor and meaning that would otherwise not exist.

In sharing these insights with others, we create communities and cultures that can sustain us through the changes and transitions of our evolving world. The richness and depth of our experience is diminished to the degree that we ignore or discount our inner life.

We can take our cues and clues to regaining this lost dimension from the actions and expressions of our younger friends and especially our Inner Child. Our next group of activities will offer opportunities to access this inner level of reality so that we can draw on its powers and perspectives to enhance the joy we find in life as a whole.

We have been playing with our senses, with toys, and with the elements. Let's consider now how we might play with words, images, and feelings. . . .

Finding Our Way Home

The Guided Replay we went through earlier is an excellent example of just such an exercise. By tapping into the memories and feelings of our early life, we can rejuvenate the experience of our present one. You may wish to revisit your childhood more often to recover the riches that remain there.

A Blueprint for Play

Some people find it fun to draw a blueprint of their childhood home or homes. Using their memories, old photos, and family members as guides, they draw out a floor plan of the place they lived at a certain age, then they mark on the plan what their fondest memories were of each room and the ways they used to play in them. (Don't forget the attic, the basement, the hall closet, the garage— all those spaces your parents didn't know you played in.)

We recommend you keep your focus on the positive for this exercise, and let anything else that shows up go by for now. The other things that happened are important too, but if you find yourself feeling worse rather than better as you do this activity, that is just a sign that you could use some experienced support as you move back to reclaim the world of your childhood. As mentioned earlier, the work of John Bradshaw and others is especially helpful in such cases, and a support group, counselor, or therapist can be priceless.

A Pleasure Map

More ambitious players can do the same with the surrounding neighborhood as well. Given the range of play behaviors, one could make a map that locates the treasures of pleasure that were discovered, created, and explored as a child. The secret hideouts, the vacant lots, the schoolyard hangouts, the haunted house. The back forty, the nearby creek, the places you played hide and seek.

There are even ways to age the resulting map by rumpling the paper and soaking it in weak coffee so that it has all of the ambience of a long-lost, honest-to-goodness Pleasure Map. (Test out your techniques first on some practice maps, we don't want your finished version to disintegrate before your very eyes.) Then you could hide it in an inaccessible part of your play journal that is protected by a secret password known only to you (and a few other trusted members of your crew). Allow yourself to re-enter the world of your childhood, and you create a universe of memory in which your Inner Child will play.

A delightful and sensitive guide for this type of replay is the book by Christopher Biffle, *A Journey Through Your Childhood*. Through its words, drawings, and imagery work, you can begin the long, perilous, and ultimately enriching adventure of recapturing your own experience of childhood.

The Hero's and Heroine's Journey

Another use of our imaginative skills can come as we find a new way to understand and share the story of our life. At some point in the past, we have all had someone tell us stories. Many of us have passed along the favor by telling stories to children in our turn.

Few pleasures are as exquisite as the ones that came along with a marvelous adventure story told to us by someone we loved as we cuddled up in his or her lap in a rocking chair.

We can create some of that same energy now by gathering up our Inner Child, imagining a peaceful, pleasant setting, and telling the story of our life as if it were a fable from once upon a time.

Use your imagination as you tell your story. Fill it with mysteries and magic, challenges and quests, surprises, setbacks, and successes. Tell about the things that were not as they seemed, the trials and tests undergone, and the lessons learned. Mention the unexpected allies, the unsuspected enemies, and the unrecognized resources of knowledge and power that were eventually discovered.

Remember that heroes and heroines come in an amazing range of shapes, sizes, and ages. Since the story is not yet completed, you are free to fill in the ending as you would wish it to be.

Begin your story with the phrase, "Once upon a time there was a child who . . ." Don't worry if you forget some parts, your Inner Child already knows the story anyway. It is his or her favorite one.

In fact, you may want to write the story down in your play journal so that you can remember it better, improve upon it as you figure out how, and have it to read to your children (or someone else's) someday.

A Letter from a Child

Another way to play with the words from within is to give voice to your Inner Child by helping him or her to write a letter to *you*!

Earlier in the New Game Plan you had an opportunity to write a letter to your Inner Child, conveying some of the awareness, insight, and intention you now have regarding this important part of your life. Whether you have done that yet or not, this could be a good time to extend the same possibility to your Inner Child.

By tuning in to your Inner Child in whatever way feels best to you, by releasing any need to control the outcome, and by writing out the message with your nondominant hand (the one you *don't* normally write with), you may begin to dialogue more directly with your imagination.

Begin the letter ''To My Growing-up Self . . .'' and pay attention to what the creative, childlike energy within you has to say to you now. Be sure to write it down as it comes; the struggle that will entail is part of the process of entering the world of the child. Let go of your expectations and allow yourself to be patient, this message may be different from any you would anticipate.

If this seems too difficult, then just write down what you ''imagine'' your Inner Child would say *if* you had one who decided to write.

By all means add whatever comes to your play journal for future reference.

For those who wish to do more work of this kind, we wholeheartedly recommend the books by Lucia Capacchione, particularly the one titled *Recovery of Your Inner Child*. This warm and perceptive book is a practical guide to the wonders and wisdom of our own inner self.

The rewards are not limited to gifts from the past, however. We can just as easily fly into the future to create a world-to-come as we would most desire it to be.

This moment—the age we live in—may be the only time there is, but that does not preclude us from experiencing it in the most rewarding way possible. And what if it is only one time among many?

My Perfect Playday

One delightful way we can exercise our imagination is to write down our own version of a perfect playday. Using your play journal or some blank sheets of paper, spend the next few minutes reflecting on what you could imagine to be a perfect playday set sometime in the future.

Give yourself full measure of freedom to make this day, all of it, just exactly as you would want it to be without regard to the normal limits we find ourselves bound to. You have infinite resources, unlimited friends of the appropriate quality and nature, and full access to any part of the universe in which you might desire to play. Any limitations will be strictly self-imposed.

When you finish the first draft, we have some questions for you to consider as a way of deepening your experience of this form of play. It helps immensely if you will do the writing before continuing the reading. We understand the desire to move on, but that may be just another way of resisting the very transformation you are hoping to achieve. It doesn't have to be *The* Perfect Playday, just *A* Perfect Playday.

This is *your* dream, take all of the time you need to explore it, expand it, transform it, and transcribe it. Do it now. . . .

* * *

Now that you have actually written something down (we are not above some subtle guilt-tripping when it suits our purposes), we would like you to reflect on your perfect day, answering the following questions to see what else comes up as a result.

What did you notice about your energy and emotional level as you played with the possibilities?

How easy or difficult was this exercise for you?

What limitations were the easiest to let go of?

Which ones were the hardest?

What messages did you say to yourself or feel as you went beyond your normal limitations in search of pleasure?

How did you determine when it was time to stop?

How satisfied are you with the results so far?

In what ways can you bring some element or dimension of that perfect playday into your life even now, given the realistic limitations and boundaries you must honor?

Many times the limitations we experience are those we impose upon ourselves through habit, ignorance, routine, and resignation. We have learned enough times that our desires are not going to get met and we adjust accordingly.

While this can be an essential survival strategy and one that is very appropriate at times, we may forget that times and circumstances change and new options open up as others close down.

Breaking free of our expectations, allowing our attitudes

to shift, and expanding our notion of the possible are at the heart of the process of continued growth and change that we managed so well as children. We can do so again.

If you are experiencing less than the satisfaction you desire as you attempt this exercise, you may need to ask for help. Your Inner Child, waiting for your invitation to return, might be a perfect playmate to help you to come up with a Perfect Playday.

Many more games and activities that we could do draw on the world of words and ideas as their source. We could do other fantasy stories, write ridiculous verse, make up puns, figure out jokes to go with punch lines, or come up with alternative captions for cartoons.

We will leave the choices up to you, however. For those of you who would like to play more with language and writing, we recommend *Writing the Natural Way*, by Gabriele Rico, and *Writing Down the Bones*, by Natalie Goldberg.

Imagery for the Inner Journey

We can also build on the exploratory play we did earlier with colors and forms by creating images that reflect the realities of our present life as well as the past and future.

One fascinating approach to the use of our inner knowing as a guide to our continued growth is called psychosynthesis. Originally developed by Roberto Assagioli, it is most beautifully presented in a book by Piero Ferrucci titled *What We May Be*. The next exercise is an adaptation of one from psychosynthesis.

A Shield of Power

First spend some time playing around as we suggested with the medium of your choice—oil pastels, watercolor markers, or whatever. You may not be an "artist," but you don't have to be. This will be an adventure in self-discovery. Be aware of any negative judgments that arise and tell yourself you are not here to meet anyone else's standards, just your own.

Then on an extra-large clean piece of paper, draw a circle that fills the space on the page. Divide the circle into quarters by drawing a line down the center from top to bottom and one across the center from side to side.

Then take some moments to clear your mind and relax. Allow yourself to imagine a blank screen in your mind. On that screen ask for an image to appear that represents *your life as it is right now*. Without forcing or pushing, as if you were just a neutral observer, consider your life now and allow to become clear that image or set of images that best represents how you see yourself and your circumstances.

There is no need to rush, wait until something that feels right comes along. It may be only an abstract set of colors and shapes, or it may be some specific images of what is important to you now. When you are ready, use the colors you have at hand and put those images down on the paper in the top left quadrant of the circle.

After you have completed that picture, let it dissolve in your mind and go back to the blank screen again. This time ask for an image to appear that represents *the next step or stage of your life*, one about to emerge. Look for something that embodies the direction in which you are headed as you continue your growth and development. Give yourself plenty of time to sense where you are going at this time and what is coming to fruition next.

As you are ready, draw that image in the upper right quadrant of the circle. Again, when you are finished, let that image go and come back to that clear screen you began with.

The third image to ask for is one that will represent for you *the blocks or barriers that stand in the way* of your moving to the next stage of your life. Let yourself sense—in color, shape, or patterns—those things holding you back or diverting you from the directions and purposes you see ahead. By acknowledging and identifying our barriers to growth, we are less likely to be controlled or subverted by them.

Let these blocks take shape in some image, rather than in words. Draw it in the lower left quadrant of the circle. After drawing in the blocks or barriers imagery, let that also dissolve and disappear from your mind.

Once again returning to the empty screen, ask for one final image representing *the strengths, talents, resources, and skills* you have that will carry you through the blocks and allow you to complete the emerging next step in your life. Spend some minutes letting those positive elements and abilities be acknowledged and affirmed as you discover an image or images that represents them. Using the colors available, put the images that occur into the lower right quadrant of the circle.

When you have completed all of the drawings, spend some time looking back over the entire picture. What you have is a representation of your life in its process of growth and change. It is much like the shield images used by Native American cultures to signify the particular themes and elements of their life.

By studying the whole picture we can sometimes find particular images that constitute a thread or theme in our own life, a theme we might not have been aware of in quite the same way. And often we find that allowing ourselves the freedom of a playful use of color and form stimulates unanticipated and powerful, heartfelt feelings to emerge.

These can be some of the gifts we can receive from a closer relationship with the creative energies of our Inner Child.

A Mandala of the Inner Child

In much the same way, you might want to design your own personal mandala representing the power and potentials of your Inner Child.

A mandala is the generic name for a visual symbol or design, most often circular in form, used to focus attention and inspire higher levels of insight and experience. Many forms of mandalas can be found in cultures ancient and contemporary all over the world. The Rose Window in the Cathedral of Notre Dame in Paris is one famous example, and the artistic and spiritual traditions of the Orient are filled with mandalas.

You need not be an artist to create a mandala, as you can perceive by looking at the spontaneous drawings of young children. All it takes is some openness to the imagery of shape and color and a growing sense of the meaning they have for you.

Once again, begin by relaxing into a quiet, centered space and focus on the energy you associate with your Inner Child. Concentrate on the power and purity of that curious, creative, wondering child who resides within. Allow the experience to develop slowly as colors and forms begin to emerge and move through your imagination. Try not to control the outcome; become instead a fair witness to what is happening.

When you are fully ready, use the colors you have before you to create a symbol for the energy and dynamism of your Inner Child.

Any of these or other forms of imagery work can become revelations, from our deepest sense of Self, that serve our greater interaction and engagement in the world.

For those wishing to go further with the use of art and drawing for personal enjoyment, we recommend Betty Edwards' book *Drawing on the Right Side of the Brain*. Her book is an excellent tool to help us appreciate the artistic side of our nature even if we didn't know we had one.

Feeling Free

Finally, we can also use our imaginative powers to get a feel for what it is to be a child again. Since some people are better at sensing or feeling things than they are at hearing or seeing them, this exercise might be another way for them to connect directly with the child within.

Growing Young

This guided relaxation exercise is best done in a quiet, calm setting where you will not be disturbed. You may wish to sit in a comfortable chair or lie down on the floor as you listen to the instructions. Either have a friend read them to you or create your own tape with soothing background music to guide you through the steps.

Begin by looking around the room and seeing it clearly. Then, gently closing your eyes, imagine what you just saw. Recall the objects, shapes, and colors that surround you as you sit or lie there, relaxing. . . .

In a similar way, with your eyes still closed, bring your attention to the sounds that surround you. Notice the loud ones, soft ones, those at a distance, those that come and go. . . .

Then, continuing to relax with your eyes closed, move your attention to the sensations you are experiencing as you sit in your chair or lie on the floor. Notice the feeling of your clothes against your skin, your body upon the chair or the floor, the rhythmic rise and fall of your chest as you take another deep, slow breath.

Notice any places of tightness or tension in your body. Gently, slowly, shift your position until you feel settled, comfortable, and at ease.

* * *

Now bring your awareness to your feet. Notice how they feel at the moment, even as you relax them further. Then imagine them flexing, changing, growing younger, becoming the feet of a young child—active, moving, light, free. . . . Standing on tip-toe to gain a better view . . . sliding in socks over cool, tile floors . . . curling with pleasure into the soft, green grass of spring.

Imagine all the ways your feet could play as a child. Splashing in mud puddles . . . sinking into sandpiles . . . slipping into dress-up clothes . . . swinging high into a cloud-filled sky. . . . Let your shoelaces wander . . . your socks sprout holes . . . your toes search out the one warm place between the clean, cold sheets of winter.

Give yourself all the time you need now to welcome once again the energy of the young into your feet, the feet of your Inner Child.

When you are ready, bring your attention to your legs, letting the slow, gentle tide of relaxation fill them with warmth. Then, as before, let them limber up, lighten, lift in anticipation as the energy of the child begins to flow into them as well . . . Stretching, running, skipping, climbing. . . . Push against the pedals . . . kick against the ball . . . leap into the water . . . form a cradle for a doll.

Rolling down the hillsides . . . hiding in the dark . . . let your legs carry you once more into the park. . . . Take whatever time you need now to grow young again, flexible and strong, feeling the power of your legs, the legs of your Inner Child.

When you are ready, bring your awareness up through your body, into your arms and down into your hands. Relax into them as you take a deep, slow breath. Then feel the transformation, the change begin again, let yourself remember the reach and grasp of the young child as that energy follows your thought. Swing from swaying branches . . . hug your favorite pet . . . dress the dolls and mind the store and get the table set. . . . *Wrestle with your buddies or defend yourself with sword . . . color, draw, and cut up things . . . . above all, don't get bored.*

Give yourself time now to let the awesome, energetic, unending activity of the young child enter into your upper body, arms, and hands, the body, arms, and hands of your Inner Child.

As you feel ready, finally bring your attention to your neck, your head, and into your face. Allow the relaxation to flow into all their parts. As you relax, notice the shift beginning here as well. Savor the gradual sharpening of your senses . . . the sounds, sights, and flavors of your world, the world of the young child. Feel your face brightening, your cares lifting, your smile growing . . . listen as you hum that nameless tune . . . tell that silly joke . . . laugh that incomparable, lilting, lighthearted laugh. . . . Once again take time to touch, taste, smell, hear, and see the world with the curiosity, wonder, confusion, and delight of the young child, with the sense and senses of your own Inner Child.

Allow yourself now and for the next few moments to resonate as fully as you can with the radiant, transforming, creative energy of the child within, rediscovering and recovering the experience of life becoming its own reward.

As you reconnect with the Inner Child, listen to, and pass along to the child within you, some of the messages that are appropriate for all children to hear from those who love them:

    I'm glad you are here . . .

    You are unique and precious to me . . .

    I like to be with you . . .

    I will protect and care for you . . .

    It's OK for you to move out into the world, to explore, to feel, and to be taken care of . . .

    You can do things and be supported at the same time . . .

    You can express your feelings to me as you feel them . . .

    It's OK to take the initiative, be yourself, and test your power . . .

You can trust and honor your thoughts and feelings . . .
You can learn and grow as long as you wish . . .
You are special to me just the way you are . . .
It's all right to go out on your own . . .
You are welcome to come home again . . .
I love you.

When it feels right, slowly find yourself sitting again in the chair or stretched out on the floor, in this room, gently shifting and stretching as you take a deep, full breath. Recognize the sounds and sensations of this body, this time, and, as you are ready, gently open your eyes, feeling alert, refreshed, and renewed. Welcome back. Welcome home.

How did you like growing young? If you would like to explore more of this sort of guided visualization work, many relaxation and imagery tapes and books are available for you to try out. Tapes of this and all the other guided visualizations from the New Game Plan for Recovery are available through Playmakers if you wish to make use of them, but making your own can be the best gift of all.

As outlined in his book *Focusing*, Eugene Gendlin has developed an approach that impressively uses this sort of ''felt-sense'' as a means to greater self-understanding and growth. It is a simple and powerful tool we can use to become more aware of and attuned to the wisdom of our body-knowing.

We hope you have explored and enjoyed some of these forms of inner play, but for many they are difficult indeed. Not all children had a lot of fun, and not all play remained pleasurable. In this next section we will touch on the troubles some people have had and may still have as they attempt to play.

Abuses of Play

It may seem strange to focus on abuse in a book about play. For those who have difficulty in playing, however, or even thinking about playing, it may be an essential area to explore.

Our feelings about the discomforts and dangers of play, alluded to in earlier chapters, are the result of lessons we learned as we were growing up. Under the guise of play many destructive things have been done by one person to another. The fact that these situations and experiences were not truly examples of play does not make them any easier to let go of and move beyond. The residual effects of inappropriate behavior, especially when it looks like play, can be very long-lasting.

Here we will briefly explore the darker side of "play" to reveal potential misuses and abuses of this powerful force.

It is important to remember that our fears and anxieties about becoming more playful may be *valid* responses to situations from the past that were, in spite of appearances, not truly play in the first place. When in the present we experience interactions that remind us of those times, we naturally respond with reluctance and resistance.

Much though we would wish it to be different, we may find ourselves recalling times of pain in the midst of experiences of pleasure. It is natural to question ourselves in such situations and to wonder if there isn't something wrong with us. When we can't identify or acknowledge those past experiences, they continue to affect our present life in particularly confusing ways.

Recovery is the process of recognizing such distortions, acknowledging and releasing our feelings about the events that caused them, and clarifying the differences between healthy and unhealthy behaviors so that we do not continue those patterns in the future. Finding, through experience, that there *are* safe, rewarding ways to play—*and* supportive playmates—is an important aspect of renewal, growth, and change.

To the degree that you discover unwanted feelings, memories, and sensations as you allow yourself to relax into play, remember that there *are* ways to resolve them and that their presence may be part of the healing process you are initiating. Do not hesitate to seek out help and support as you feel a need for them so that you can free the energy of your Inner Child for your continued growth.

We will look at three general ways in which play can be distorted in a destructive way. Whatever the intention, when "play" results in harm to others, to oneself, or when it is pressed into the service of an unhealthy and destructive lifestyle, it ceases to be play. Where fear, anxiety, threat, and pain exist, play is absent.

Taking Pains to Stop

While accidents can happen anytime, even in the midst of play, it is clear that play stops in such cases until the one who is hurt is taken care of or is ready to go on. When such is not the case, when people are hurt physically, emotionally, or socially, then we are no longer in the province of play.

It is a clear abuse of the play relationship to harm, humiliate, demean, devalue, or control another person or group of people. Examples abound of these unfortunate occurrences among children and adults alike. Often the abuse is hard to identify even by the one being abused.

Overzealous roughhousing is not uncommon. Each of us has probably been at some time or another the victim of inappropriate physical interaction. Despite our signals to the contrary, the other person just kept on going to the point where we may have been totally out of breath, out of control, or in actual pain. More than one incident in a swimming pool comes to mind.

The problem was that we couldn't find a way to communicate that we had stopped playing and were struggling to survive. If the error was acknowledged and the behavior changed, then no lasting harm may have been done. It was when the same thing happened too intensely or too often that our basic sense of trust became damaged and we rightfully avoided putting ourselves in that position again.

Excessive tickling is another example of misusing play. What may start out as a mutually rewarding interaction can turn into a frightening and humiliating one. There are few frustrations as great as being genuinely upset or angry only to be forced into continued laughter by inappropriate tickling. And intense laughter can put one in doubt about being able to breathe as powerfully as being held under water too long.

Emotional pain can also be a result of unhealthy approaches to play. We even have a term for it—we "make fun of someone." When anyone becomes the object of derision, humiliation, harassment, or teasing, even in a "humorous" way, the play relationship is immediately destroyed and long-term damage to one's self-image is possible.

To play one must feel safe. When our behavior causes others to have doubts for their safety, worth, or competence, we are engaged in a misuse of play.

Often a child's natural desire to play has been inappropriately limited by social sanctions and pressures in the form of gender, class, racial, or skill-level discrimination and stereotyping. Many times it is just the way a person looks or moves that marks him or her as an outcast. The pain and despair of such situations goes deep into the heart of the child.

While social standing and peer acceptance are certainly a focus of certain stages and types of play, there is an acknowledged bond that must be present for the play to continue. The moment someone is truly excluded from participation in some mutually satisfying way, they can experience a real loss of validation and connection, one of the more powerful and devastating punishments known to humankind. The depth of the rejection explains why some children will go to practically any lengths to remain included in the play.

Disparate Diversions

We are not immune to misusing play on ourselves, either. When we choose to use play as a way to divert, deny, cover up, or avoid uncomfortable or painful feelings and situations, we do harm to ourselves.

Reading may be an excellent and positive pastime. Sports may be a healthy means for generating energy and enthusiasm. Spending time with friends can be renewing and rewarding. When any of these activities becomes an excuse to avoid important responsibilities or ignore commitments to ourselves or others, however, we are in danger of causing more problems than we currently have.

It is largely a question of balance in such situations. When anything comes to dominate our life, even "play," we have to be careful or we are headed for a fall.

We can also sometimes stumble by confusing fantasy with illusion. In our desire to maintain a relationship, accomplish a goal, or acquire a prized object, we may fool ourselves along the way.

Fantasy is a marvelous outlet for the imagination, and often a means to affirming new possibilities. But when we can no longer distinguish between imagination and reality, we are lost in an illusion, and vulnerable to that which we cannot see.

If our desire to have or keep something or someone is

so great that we no longer perceive the price of our perseverance, we are putting ourselves at risk in an unbal-
anced and unhealthy way. Regardless of the apparent
prize, we are no longer at play.

Captivating Pastimes

Finally, we need to address the unique situation where
"play" is used in the service of a compulsive disease. We
have all met persons for whom "party" is a verb. Though
they may be delightful, charming companions to a point,
it soon becomes obvious that the party is more important
than the people, and the charm has a life span shorter
than we expected.

Drinking or drugging excessively is often associated
with "having a good time." The unfortunate fact is that
for some persons the results can be equivalent to a slow-
motion suicide, the exact opposite of life-enhancing play.

There are other forms of compulsive behavior that on
the surface look like play. When gambling, high-risk
sports, and sexual behaviors become dangerous to the
health and welfare of the practitioner *or* others, however,
they have no place in the world of play.

Of course, an authentic experience of play is an element
essential to recovery as an addiction is recognized, acknowledged, and interrupted. The theme of this chapter
and of the entire book is that the genuine experience of
play *is* a healing force in the process of recovery and the
experience of life.

Relearning to play may require us to confront again
some of the wounds we received early in life, but the
potential for resolution and recovery from those wounds
is present as well. In safe, satisfying, and secure settings,
we can *recontact* the energy of the Inner Child, *renew* the
relationship that has been with us since our very beginning, and *reclaim* the positive power of play and make it
ours for keeps.

6

Partners in Play

Laughter is the shortest distance between two people.
VICTOR BORGE

As part of the basic New Game Plan, we had you take a look at your Play Community. These are the people you recognize as your regular (or potential) playmates in your "Play Management Program." We would like to expand on that initial step in this section to focus your attention on the ways in which play can not only help you to feel better about life, but improve the quality of your relationships as well.

The sad fact is that often we tend to fall into all-too-familiar patterns when relating to the very people we care about most. After all, when someone achieves the status of "family" (familiar), he or she becomes a part of us in a more permanent sort of way and we may end up taking him or her for granted. This is not what any of us would

wish to have happen to us or to anyone else; it just seems
to occur without our being aware of it.

Can you think of someone you feel neglected by? (We
considered making this following section **off limits** to our
wives and children, but that would do us no good. They
already know us too well.) Is there anyone you may be
taking for granted? (At least *we* have good excuses. There
is this book to write and our jobs to keep up with and the
lawn to mow and some volunteer work we plan to start
soon and—It's no use, we have *no* excuse. We, too, have
some playing to do.) Are there people in your life you
would like to get closer to in a mutually satisfying way?
There probably are. How about setting up some playtime
together?

One old saying has it that if we could treat our friends
and family more like we treat new acquaintances and treat
new acquaintances more like family, the world would be
a better place. There's some truth there, and we want to
help you take advantage of it.

Think back to the time you first met your current partner or close friend or work buddy. Many times in the
development of a deep friendship or relationship there is
a time of real delight and joy along the way. Do you recall
some special moments (or days, weeks, months) with this
important person in your life? What were you doing during those times?

Our hunch is that as you developed the close bond that
sustains you now, you found (and made) lots of opportunities to play together. Remember what that was like?

Make a brief list of the rewarding, enjoyable, satisfying
things you used to do with each other. When was the last
time you did any of those things on a regular basis? (You
don't have to answer that last question out loud. . . .)

Don't despair. Even if it has been an awfully long
time, or you can't even remember what *was* fun back

then, remember, IT'S NEVER TOO LATE TO HAVE A HAPPY . . .

What about now? Can you imagine a playful way to spend some time together? Pretend you are planning a date or a long weekend. How could you organize an honest-to-goodness, old-fashioned, rip-roaring good time?

Our special advisors on healthy relationships assure us this is the way to go. (And they also have given us just *one more chance* to start walking our talk!) The funny part is that it can be great for everyone involved.

How come we work so hard to avoid having a good time?

One problem we have run into from time to time is that our planning process is not working the way it should. We have been in the groove so long it has become a rut. We find ourselves automatically hauling out the same stale old options for spending the evening or day together. Anything you try for too long loses its punch. If it's important to enliven even a well-adjusted, comfortable, and somewhat predictable relationship—and it *is* important—we have to create some new possibilities for playing.

How about generating a Wish List? Talk to your friend, partner, spouse, or the spice of your life (not a bad way to start, in any case, especially if you haven't found much time for that lately), and give him or her a copy of our genuine, customized, patented—

Wish List

As part of your program to have more friendship, fun, and life in your life, please fill out the following sections of this wish list. (For those of you with a completed Fun List, this should be a breeze. For the majority of you, get to work!) Feel free to modify, magnify, or manipulate the form to make it serve you.

1. How many ways can you think of to have fun for free with a friend? List at least fifteen. _____

_____

2. What are some things you could do to have fun with a friend that cost less than $25 each? List several. _____

_____

3. What do *I* think my special friend would like to do together with me? List at least five. _____

_____

4. What are some fun things to do that my friend probably *hasn't* thought of yet? List three. _____

_____

5. What could we do together for fun by next week? ____

_____

6. What am I willing to do for sure by this weekend? ____

_____

7. What could we do starting now? _____

_____

Be sure your friend fills one of these out and *you* fill one out, *then* sit down to compare your results. From that base of information, start planning what you *will* do together to have some fun soon. A suggestion is to shy away from the things you already do on a fairly regular basis. Break some new ground—or at least hike over it!

Do two fun things a week for a month and come back to see us. Your relationship should be noticeably healthier by then.

You are aware by now, perhaps, that we aren't talking magic here. This is no mysterious, high-priced cure for all that "ails ya." We would have a hard time stretching this into a hot new best-seller for the relationship market. (We tried, but the editor had better sense.)

No, the reality we are faced with is that our meaningful, intimate relationships blossom only when we feed them. And the brightest colors come along when the lightest feelings are included in our daily interactions. It's a fairly simple proposition (except in practice).

In order to facilitate this process taking place, we have made special arrangements with a major financial institution to bring you the latest tool for relationship enhancement. You have been preapproved for charter membership in the Recover Card program!

Features include a high interest rate compounded daily, monthly statements of utilization, no annual fees, guaranteed satisfaction, and only positive credit reports allowed. And you get something back *each time you use it*! (Think what happens when you use the other cards.)

The plan is simple, painless, and designed to take away any excuse for delaying gratification for you and your friends beyond a reasonable interval. It's all part of our "play as you go" plan.

Here's how it works. You sign up with a good friend, partner, or buddy using the handy Recover Card we have included on the next page. (Feel free to buy another book or contact us at Playmakers if you have more than one friend.) By giving them the card, you are assuring your

RecoverCard

The card that backs your play.

Recover your sense of hope,
　　　　your sense of joy,
　　　　　　your sense of humor.

Discover play as the way life becomes
its own reward.

_____

Signature of Issuer

full backing in an extended line of play credits for use as opportunities and interest arise.

You see, many people have not yet set up their Play Money program and may be out of usable cash for purely pleasurable purposes just when they think of something fun they could do with you. By using their Recover Card, they have the right to contact you even if they can't quite cover the cost in order to find out if you have the time, money, and interest to pick up the remaining tab.

As the issuer of the card, you have the right and responsibility to be completely honest in either accepting the offer, modifying it to a suitable extent, or making a counteroffer for some future date. You can rest assured that as you accrue play credits by consenting to the invitation, you will be able to redeem them in return with increased interest at your preferred time and place.

Once a month at a minimum, there will be a joint auditing conference where the two of you get together to

Principles of Play:
1. Play is not for real (but it is real fun!)
2. When you can do so safely, suspend judgment (and fear of judgment) in favor of fun.
3. Put process before product.
4. Put some imagination into your challenges.
5. Do it..............differently!

The bearer of this card is hereby authorized to request play time from the issuer of the card whenever desired. Bearer agrees to extending play credits in return when circumstances and interests permit.

For further information consult: <u>The New Game Plan for Recovery,</u> Tobin Quereau and Tom Zimmermann, Ballantine Books 1992.

assess the success of the program and set up plans to balance out the accounts. You are allowed at that time to make any positive reports to each other's credit and reaffirm the agreement for the next period.

Be sure to offer the card only to the person or persons who qualify by your rigorous standards. This is an exclusive opportunity that should be offered only to your most preferred applicants. (And, as you know from experience, they don't have to be aware of the program in advance to be considered applicants.) Just be sure that they are willing partners in the agreement so that the interest rate will be at its highest level possible during the term of the agreement.

If you will follow a regular program of reinvesting your play credits as soon as you accumulate them, your relationship should grow stronger, more rewarding, and more mutually satisfying.

When our Inner Child can play with someone else's,

we are bonding at levels of vulnerability, openness, trust, and joy that are hard to match any other way. At these levels, the message that we value and care about them is conveyed in unmistakable ways. In play, giving and receiving pleasure are one.

That's worth something, isn't it?

The Family That Plays Together, Stays Together

All the more reason not to forget our family along the way. While none of the above excludes kids, the tone is decidedly on the adult level. We want to remind you to carry that energy also into your relationships with your children as well, if you have any. (If not, import some, they are great excuses to give your Inner Child a shot at some longed-for play.)

While, in general, one might assume that the children in a family will automatically insure plenty of opportunity for play, in reality their insistence is rarely enough. Our behavior as adults has a lot to do with the modeling we received when we were children, and, unfortunately, many of us did not perceive our parents as being very playful very much of the time.

Adding to the difficulty for some adults is the fact that they can't even remember *themselves* as having been very playful as *children*! The various events, situations, and pressures that block their memory of early years also puts their positive experiences of play beyond reach for now. How then, without help, can they expect to do much for their children? As adults most of us must relearn the art of playing as (and with) a child. What better teachers than our children themselves?

The operating principle here will be to take the cues

from the child while taking care of ourselves in the process. As a suggestion for where to start, we will discuss briefly some of the developmental aspects of childhood play; that will give you some further guidelines for good times (and some assistance in recall for those who could use it).

Again, the planning process is important. We aren't suggesting that you plan your spontaneity, rather that you plan in some *time* for it. You value doing the dirty laundry enough to fit it into every week. How about cleaning up your act with your kids on a regular basis as well? They will outgrow those clothes in no time at all, but you can't buy more time with them from a store.

For more details on the developmental aspects of play, we refer you to a marvelous book by Brian and Shirley Sutton-Smith called *How to Play with Your Children (and when not to)*. It may be hard to find, but it is worth it.

Infants

Play starts when we do. Even infants at the earliest of ages find ways to playfully explore their bodies, their companions, and the environment around them. Since they are fairly immobile for a time, we need to be more active in providing them opportunities for interaction and exploration.

In their first few months of life, children are most eloquent with their bodies, particularly their mouths. Lots of games can be generated just by actively searching out what stimulates them to pay attention and respond with energy. Although smiles often take a few weeks to appear in profusion, even with newborns close observation usually can indicate whether they are having a good time or not.

Reflection and amplification seem to be the key concepts here. Take what you see them doing and make it bigger. Help them to stretch a bit and feel the pleasure of confirmation and validation for their effort. Make a face no one could ignore and see if they ignore you. Create sounds unheard of in human experience, and see if they can top them (don't forget, that's what they do all day long). Peek a "boo" between your fingers and be prepared for any reaction. If you are acting sufficiently foolish to hope no other adult is within five miles who could possibly report you to the authorities, you are probably on the right track.

The power of an infant's gaze is immense: If they are locked on and learning, you will know it! And then there is the fail-safe mechanism all children come equipped with called a "cry." They waste no time letting you know if you are headed in the *wrong* direction with your play. For people who can't talk, they are marvelously eloquent communicators.

Pay attention to your own energy level as well as the child's. When *either* one of you looks restless or feels tired of the action, take a break. Short doses of love and attention on a frequent basis are generally the most appropriate. Remember, if it isn't fun for you, the message you want to convey is probably not going to be communicated anyway.

Toddlers

Now we are into real action. These little tykes are faster than a speeding parent, more maneuverable than an aging uncle, and able to fall over anything in a single bound. They can yank, push, stuff, drag, and hide incredible amounts of supposedly safe valuables in the time it takes to turn your back. And they suddenly grow much less tolerant of interfering adults. For a variety of reasons, not the least of which are enumerated above, a primary addition to the repertoire of infants is the generic "chase."

With very little encouragement, toddlers figure out that in order to remain free they must learn how to flee, and this natural motivation is the foundation for numerous fast-moving forms of chase. After some practice as escape artists, the toddlers may try out their hand at the attack mode and delight in "scaring" anyone and everyone willing to cower and scatter in fear.

A suitable termination to the game of chase is, of course, the horseplay that comes upon capture. Grabbing, tickling (within limits), hugging, swinging, and even devouring are called for repeatedly (just be sure they *are* being called for—too much of this sort of thing falls under the topic we covered earlier, the abuse of play).

As toddlers grow further in age and skill, language games, songs and verses, finger play, and pretend games enter the scene. All of this is in addition to the massive amounts of just plain movement and action activities the children will initiate—such as trashing their rooms in under six seconds with one hand holding a teddy bear. Again, to the degree consistent with your own enjoyment, let them lead the way.

Three to Five Years

During these ages, kids usually get their body control and physical skill worked out to a large degree. After this time it is mostly refinement and elaboration of these abilities. There is a marvelous symmetry and grace that often occurs somewhere about this period, causing one author to describe these ages as "the magical years." The body catches up to the head and the mind matches up with the muscles in a way that is a delight to see. (Even the kids usually realize by this time that they know it all, and demand treatment equal to that accorded all the *other* grownups in the house.)

In addition to the inevitable outdoor action activities, storytelling becomes more elaborate and complex. Pretend conversations with dolls, telephones, or pets are extensive. Simple board and card games become manageable. Art activities are more sophisticated as children learn to handle drawing, finger-painting, coloring, and cutting. Building elaborate structures may become a fad, with the destruction of them a close second in preference. (Cleaning them up remains dead last.)

Social games and interactions are more the focus now, replacing the "parallel play" of the two-year-old. Imitation and role plays become more elaborate and sustained. "Pretend" is the password to limitless pleasure—"You be the dog and I'll be the Mommy!" Word games, songs, and rhyming are big, with outlandish distortions of the "normal" delivery guaranteed to elicit laughter. "Happy Birthday to lamp" (and to chair, ceiling, etc.) is good for several minutes of silliness.

Secrets, surprises, and social rituals make regular appearances, and being someone's "best friend" is as much a currency to be bargained with as a commitment to undying affection.

Fools are still tolerated and exaggeration is acceptable within limits, but reality is closing in fast, and a "silly Daddy" can sometimes be the object of scorn as well as delight. Children by this age are consummate realists, reflecting all too accurately our personal and societal habits. "Do as I say, not as I do," was first said by an exasperated parent to a five-year-old. (The child replied passionately, "That's not fair!")

Six and Seven

Improvisation is a key addition to play with this age group. Along with the continuing expansion and elaboration of physical skills, with all the associated running, riding, climbing, catching, swinging, sliding, and trashing of rooms, children are more apt to improvise rather than just imitate. Pursuit and escape become neighborhood-wide phenomena, and bike-riding becomes the bane of many a traffic-wise parent.

Children may *demand* to have playmates now, when not

long before, solitary play was a regular option and parents were a suitable substitute for a friend. With proper behavior an adult will still do in a pinch, but only when appropriate protocol is followed and a sincere attitude toward play is demonstrated.

Especially with the advent of school, relationships with other children often take on significant new levels of importance. Learning about inclusion and rejection is a central part of their lives, even in their play. Who gets to play and what they play are the subject of great debate.

The roles of Mommy and Daddy, kings and queens, cops and robbers are more finely drawn and longer lasting than at earlier ages. Though characters from television may replace the heroes from fairy tales, the investment in the roles is similar and just as essential to the play. "Let's pretend" still announces hours of activity, interrupted only by "unnecessary" mealtimes and unwilling partners—"I *always* have to be the boy! You *never* let me be the girl. I'm going home unless . . . ."

Eight to Thirteen

From here on out, the range and sophistication of play is extensive. Largely comfortable on their own and often out of sight, children are able to build with both their hands and their imaginations, constructing far-reaching fantasies as easily as the neighborhood fort.

As they learn to manage rules and rituals with greater skill, games of all sorts—board games, sandlot sports, street games, pretend games, games of chance, card games—fill up their days and nights with challenge. Competition becomes more blatant and control often a factor as abilities are tested against the force of gravity and the face of an opponent.

By this time, especially when encouraged by status-conscious schools and parents, scores may become more important than skills, and we see the long, slow transition from play to performance begin in earnest.

Fourteen and Above

Beyond here lie dragons. . . . Given the fast-changing pattern of contemporary society and values, we will make no comments about what teenagers play with or how. If there are any teenagers in your life you are encouraged to borrow some money from them, get all the professional help you can, and double the amount of play in your own life. Perhaps that will assist with the particular stressors inherent in the condition to which you are subject. In any case, if your teenagers have developed any skill at all in make-believe by this time, you will never know *anything* about what they are really up to anyway.

You may have noticed in this all-too-brief synopsis of typical play behaviors the relative absence of the single most dominant activity engaged in by children of all ages: watching the tube. Television fills more hours of a child's life than does school, equals or exceeds in cases the time they spend with peers, and dwarfs the time spent with parents on the order of the proverbial universe and a grain of sand.

While we do have some concerns about the effects of excessive TV watching, we are mainly not focusing on television largely because it doesn't really fit in with our sense of playing. While, at times, it may inspire the imagination, instruct the intellect, and excite the emotions, it is simply too passive a pastime and too externally controlled a medium for us to link it very directly with play. We would generally prefer a pile of dirt or a vacant lot to the typical fare on most channels. (That is, unless it is a show *we* like to watch.)

But where do we find the time for all of this good play?

There's the cooking to do, the yard to mow, the laundry to wash, the reports to write, the—

The litany again.

We know, in the normal course of events there is *no* place for play. So when you can't fit in a good chunk of playtime with your kids, settle for making something playful out of the time you do have.

How can you make a game out of collecting the laundry? Who can find the most clothes to put in the laundry basket? Who can throw their clothes in the basket with one eye closed? How fast can you get the dirty clothes out of the room and into the clothes hamper?

Getting riled by someone big enough to bite you on the knee? Get really riled. Huff and puff! Make faces. Roll your eyes and growl like a giant. Make a game out of getting your frustration out in the open. As long as the little ones figure out it *is* a game, it lets you vent some anger and distracts them from whatever they were doing before. When they have entered into the game themselves, they are already cooperating with you and there is a chance you can get some positive action in the direction you would like.

Find yourself driving around the town with the young ones in tow? Use the time to sing songs (that can sound pretty funny without half trying), play rhyming games or "I Spy." Tell a story or listen to one. See who can guess the color of the next car. With older kids, see who can identify the make and model of the cars you pass. Estimate the exact arrival time for your next stop (no cheating just because you are driving). See how long the kids can hold their breath. Stop when they pass out. . . .

These are just a few suggestions, but the key is to never forget that the power of possibility in play makes anything more enjoyable—even eating peas. ("I'll bet you can't eat all of 'em one at a time.")

For those of you without children, this developmental

sketch of play behaviors need not be a total waste. You too can share some playtime with a child, by applying for designation (or appointing yourself) as an Honorary Uncle or Aunt. Most families with kids find it a necessity to extend this title to more than one aspiring candidate just to make it through the first few years.

Suitable responsibilities involve the inevitable trips to the zoo (for the seventh time this year), the park, or the swimming hole, a kite flying contest or two, instruction in the childly art of paper airplane making (and flying), birthday presents of an appropriate nature (on time), and the like.

Benefits include, but are not limited to, hugs on arrival and departure (with accompanying tears for a particularly talented performance), cards at holiday time and occasionally for no reason at all, smiles, laughter, ice cream cones that drip, immensely grateful parent(s), and strange stains on the backseat of the car that never quite come out.

Another use for this survey of play is for all of us who are seeking a better connection to the child within us who is yearning to be free. By giving ourselves some time exploring activities of the sort outlined above, whether on our own, with willing children, or even other interested adults, we may begin to create the atmosphere of support, trust, and validation that we did not experience as fully as we wished when we were growing up.

An example. Once when I (Tobin) was teaching in a preschool setting, I decided to sit down at the art table with the four-year-olds to join in on the project at hand. This was in the San Francisco Bay area, and we had been studying the upcoming Chinese New Year celebration. After a particularly interesting story about the holiday activities, the assignment was to paint a picture of a New Year's parade.

I squeezed into one of the tiny chairs, shoved my knees

under the table and set to work on a massive green dragon. I am *not* an artist. (How many of us have said *that* over the years?) My dragon began to look more like an Army duffle bag full of potatoes that were beginning to sprout than anything remotely dangerous. I struggled. I sweated. I made adjustments in my plan. (One cannot, I discovered, erase tempera paints.) I looked for excuses to leave.

The child next to me finally looked over at my efforts. I shall never forget his face. I shall never forget his picture, either. His image was aglow with life. He had splashed, flipped, thrown, and swirled an amazing array of color onto his once empty white paper. In it I could see and almost hear firecrackers exploding, people screaming in surprise and delight, bells ringing and lights flashing. Across the page, snaking its way in every direction, was a mythical beast, a dragon of the gods, half-hidden by the throng but ever-present in energy and movement.

Finally he spoke to me gently. "You know, Tobin, why your picture doesn't look too good?" I held my breath. "You never do just what you want," he said, continuing to experiment with banging his brush against his finger to watch the spray that shot onto his masterpiece (and onto the tabletop as well).

I took another look at my "dragon." It was true. I had been seduced by the *thought* of a dragon and the *effort* of "making" one. He was simply having fun with colors. My product was dull, lifeless, and ugly. His was continuing to grow even as he spoke. I felt old and embarrassed.

But I learned that day something I have never forgotten. I received a gift that continues to be given. I found that the source of pleasure is only as far away as I make it, and that I too, even as an adult, can tap into the richness of experience to find the treasures that are there for the taking. *For free.*

I crumpled up my paper and threw it gladly away. His went with the others on the bulletin board. Neither work has been forgotten—but I wish I had stolen his.

I could not have learned what I learned without entering the arena of play. In risking the outcome that so clearly occurred, I gained a lesson that had been otherwise denied. I resolved to put myself into play more directly and more often after that. I thought it to be revolutionary. The kids thought it just made good sense.

By diving into the experience and noticing which aspects and levels of play attract us and which leave us uneasy or unsettled, we may also possibly learn which parts of our Inner Child could stand attention and nourishment.

Recognizing that judgment and blame inhibit play as well as other aspects of learning and changing, we must learn to explore with a goal of acceptance and understanding in spite of the other feelings that may come along. The fact is that we have the opportunity now to do for ourselves what others could not do for us earlier. Let's make the most of it!

Creating, promoting, and allowing play into our lives and relationships is a powerful path to self-healing and recovery. The journey may seem long and sometimes dangerous, even though the goal is in sight. An active play community insures we will have companions and colleagues along the way.

7

Play Works

Imagination is more important than knowledge.
ALBERT EINSTEIN

Play is not the easiest of subjects to define or explore. It is infinite in form even if it seems to have some common themes or elements. Play may be evident to the player much more readily than it is to the observer.

One expert is reported to have said, "Studying nuclear physics is child's play compared to studying child's play." It is that very diversity of form, however, and that core of function, that makes it possible for us to discover (and recover) playful aspects to *whatever* we do—even when others would call it "work"!

The recovery of a sense of play can proceed on many levels. In our New Game Plan workshops we create an environment and an experience that helps people contact once again that powerful, playful child within each of us.

The description of child's play in the previous chapters and the prescriptions for becoming more playful focus actively on this aspect of play.

When we can re-establish a relationship with the child we were (or wanted to be) and give ourselves what we needed then, we are actively engaged in a healthy, healing process with great benefits in our present lives.

We know, however, from our own observations and from extensive research in the field, that play is not a static, stable phenomenon. As children grow their play changes, and not always because of some external force or limitation. Play changes because what *feels good* changes as we learn and grow.

In order to help us better create rewarding, renewing experiences wherever we are, at whatever age or stage, we explore now what play may look like in a more developmental sense. With this knowledge, a little practice, and some help from our friends, we can continue "growing young" *all* the days of our lives.

Just what that playful adult experience would look and feel like has been described particularly well by a man with a fascinating theory and an equally fascinating name. Dr. Mihaly Csikszentmihalyi has focused his attention and research for many years on the phenomena of play behavior in adults. His interest is in the subjective *experience of playfulness* rather than in a theory of play itself.

As a result, he and his researchers interviewed intensively hundreds of people who spent a good bit of their time in behavior that was motivated not basically by external rewards, but more by an inner satisfaction with the process itself. The initial subjects included chess masters, rock climbers, dancers, athletes. . . . From their investigations they found an amazing consistency of response as the subjects described what it felt like when things were going well for them in their "play."

Later on the researchers confirmed similar reactions

from more conventional role models such as secretaries, surgeons, teachers, assembly line workers, and managers.

It appears that the experience of choice was one that had, among others, these characteristics: a sense of *concentration* or deep involvement, described as a kind of merging of action and awareness in the moment; usually the participants reported a clear *goal* or end result that they were seeking, and *immediate feedback* on how they were doing in achieving it. The absorption was so great that often there was a sense of *time distortion*—sometimes events occurred as if in slow motion and at other times hours went by in a flash.

Accompanying all of this was a *feeling of control* or influence over events but in a curiously *egoless* way. Concern over the results or outcome did not intrude on the activity itself. Some people described it as almost a transcendent state, a *union* with the process underway. From the many responses, the term *flow* emerged as an apt descriptor for this particular blend of awareness and activity.

The responses seemed to reflect a dynamic balancing between the *challenge* in a situation and the *skills* necessary to meet it. Where the challenge was perceived as too great (or too "real"), anxiety or even fear set in. When the skills were more than adequate for the challenge, boredom ultimately appeared. There was a fairly predictable range of arousal and stimulation, which, when balanced by appropriate skilled interventions and responses, resulted in a pleasurable resolution of the tension generated in the process—"I *did* it!"

Play, from this perspective, might then be the process of maintaining the intrinsically rewarding *flow* experience for as long as desired given the environment—both internal and external—at hand.

The beauty of play is that while we are in its fold, we are simultaneously living at our edges and in touch with our center. We are in control of a situation that is beyond our control. We are exercising our abilities and extending our power, bending the world to our will.

When the play goes well we have succeeded in enlarging our reach, expanding our potential, exceeding our limitations. When things don't *flow* well we have merely added a measure of intensity and energy to the challenge with no other long-term debilitating consequences.

As Dr. Csikszentmihalyi describes it, in play we are "living at our optimal capacity."

This particular model and theory helps to explain some of the attraction people can feel in such diverse activities as fishing, hang gliding, collecting stamps, playing (and watching) sports, running, punning, and generally just messing around.

The difference between play and work is that in work, while the rewards can be as potent, the consequences are often not as benign. And unlike at play, at work we are not so likely to be in control of what happens to us or with us. Remember Tom Sawyer?

As we will see, however, those who can merge their work and play are truly blessed, having reached that delightful state of "being paid to play"!

Keeping in mind what the *flow* experience is and our earlier definition of play (a voluntary activity at once invigorating and relaxing, challenging and rewarding, unpredictable yet unthreatening, and above all a process we enjoy), let's look at how we might find play in some fairly unexpected places.

Working It Out

It should be no wonder that people often differentiate clearly between play and work. From a fairly early age we are told to "quit playing around and get to work," whether that means cleaning up our rooms, mowing the yard, or finishing our homework. Work has purpose and utility. It is a necessary part of being responsible and growing up. It fills the table and pays the bills.

The biggest trouble with work is that it often becomes an end in itself. We begin to value ourselves and others mainly by the work that we do. How many times have you ever met someone—even at a party—and been asked, "What do you *do*?" Our appearance, status, and lifestyle reflect our chosen career. We can even become addicted to the process of work and suffer severe withdrawal symptoms when we are separated from it for very long. All of this contributes to the reality of chronic stress we spoke of in the beginning of this book.

So what's there to do about it? We do *have to work, you know!* Of course we do. And most of us probably do well at it. But there is the chance that we can improve the quality of our work life *and* our performance if we actively incorporate a playful attitude into our 8-to-5 life.

Let's explore what that might look, feel, and sound like. Get set for more "work."

In order to create more enjoyment in our work life, we need to know what we already do that is particularly interesting, satisfying, and/or rewarding. Thinking about your daily (or nightly) routine, from the time you leave (or settle down) for work, what are the parts of your job that you look forward to most?

Notice whether it is the interaction with others that you especially enjoy (and with which others), or the challenge of a particularly puzzling problem that you get to respond to. Pay attention to the pacing you feel fits you best. What do you do that gets you active, energized, excited? What part of your job—however small—seems to refresh and renew you rather than just wear you out?

Fill out the rest of the following questions as you complete the exercise we call:

Uplifts

(And remember, work does not have to be *salaried* to qualify as work.)

At work I enjoy . . . _____

_____

I look forward to . . . _____

_____

My favorite activity is . . . _____

_____

My favorite time of the day is . . . _____

_____

I enjoy being around . . . _____

_____

I get a real sense of satisfaction when . . . _____

_____

I miss being able to . . . _____

_____

I'd like to be able to . . . _____

_____

It feels good when . . . _____

_____

The time goes by quickest when . . . . _____

_____

I have the most fun when . . . _____

_____

If you are now saying to yourself—*Here they go again, asking silly questions. This is WORK we are talking about! Do they think I do this for fun? That's why they have to* pay *me to come back every day!*—even so there's hope. Work, like other pastimes, does offer us opportunities for change. Since our "reality" has a lot to do with our attitudes, beliefs, and perceptions, there is always room for adjustment.

If you can't find much at all that is positive about your present work setting, what can you *imagine* might be fun? Is there some other aspect of the job you would like to be doing? Would you enjoy taking on a different set of duties and responsibilities? How would you change things around your workplace if you had some magic dust and could change it into a work*playce*? You see, the nice thing about playing around with this stuff is that you don't have to stick with just the way things are, you can try on for size how they *could be*.

Experimenting with what feels good is not just a self-centered activity, either. Research into what motivates employees to the highest levels of performance has consistently shown that, in the words of *The One-Minute Manager*, "People who feel good about themselves produce good results."

The factors that seem to be most powerful in creating good feelings and motivation in workers are appropriately challenging work, a sense of achievement, recognition for work well done, a feeling of responsibility, an experience of growth and development. Remind you of going with the *flow*?

Think how much more valuable an employee or successful a supervisor you could be if you truly enjoyed what you were doing most of the time. Whatever level of satisfaction you now feel, see if you can notice what contributes to that feeling and increase its prevalence, consistency, and intensity. Begin now. (It helps if you go back and write out a few of those silly sentences. You may notice something you have missed before.)

In addition to the basic research assignment we just made, there are some other things we can suggest that you consider as options for more enjoyment (and effectiveness) as you work. Several of them are modeled on the ideas included in an excellent book by Edward de Bono, *Lateral Thinking: Creativity Step by Step*.

A Play Management Program

USE YOUR IMAGINATION. (Ever see that before?) When it comes to routine, responsibility, and real problem solving, make use of that child-given talent for creativity that we all had at one time even if it seems sadly out of shape today.

If part of your job is a very repetitious, somewhat solitary activity, make a game of it. Challenge yourself to a race and see who wins. Keep track of your performance from one period of time to the next and see if you can find a more efficient (or fun) way to get the job done. Vary something about the way you do what you do. Handicap yourself and see if you still can perform at the same high levels with a little practice. (Don't tell your supervisor we said that!) Stretch yourself and see what happens. Reward yourself for taking a risk. Congratulate yourself for being a winner.

You might even organize teams and a tournament for all those other lonely souls who are as tired as you are of doing the same old thing. Just think: fanfares, trophies, a hall of fame! The possibilities are endless. The fun begins with you.

When you feel weighed down by responsibilities and can't seem to get the help you need, try looking at things another way. Set down on a sheet of paper your most troublesome "hassles" (we'll let you supply the paper for this one; we did the "uplifts") and then, one by one, ask yourself "WHAT'S GOOD ABOUT IT?" No kidding, we are absolutely serious about this and so is Sidney X. Shore, a creativity consultant who calls it being an "Angel's Advocate."

We all know full well how to do the opposite. We tell ourselves endlessly what is wrong with the way things are. We probably know at least a couple of other experts in the devil's advocate corps, as well. This inversion of the expected behavior, however, takes some real skill in playing with possibilities we never imagined before.

The truth of the matter is that these hassles usually are incredibly persistent (that's what makes them hassles) because there are so many reasons why they remain that we just haven't ever considered. By standing things on their heads for a while, we may uncover what contributes to their staying power and find more effective and satisfying ways to meet those particular needs.

The other benefit of being an Angel's Advocate is that,

on occasion, we may discover a whole new perspective on an important part of our job that had been covered up by the status quo. What's good about getting a new boss? She may be the one who finally listens to your wild and crazy ideas!

One other related phrase to keep in mind after you have found out *what's* good *about it*, is to USE EVERYTHING TO YOUR ADVANTAGE. Advertisers tend to be good at this. We're number two—we try harder! We *only* make copiers! Fire sale! Lost our lease! Inventory tax sale! You know the routine—when life hands you a lemon, make lemonade.

When you are loaded down with responsibilities, your other option is to try and handle them all. We have tried that. It doesn't work.

Now when you run up against *real* problems (they differ from regular problems in that you have *no* idea how the heck you are going to resolve them and you are zooming toward a deadline) there are still some things you might try. If you haven't come up with a reasonable solution and you are starting to panic, we suggest you CHALLENGE ASSUMPTIONS.

You see, most of the time when we feel pressured, trapped, or otherwise limited in untenable ways, that feeling is as much a consequence of our own assumptions as anyone else's. When we can't see our way out of a situation, it may be time to revisit the old-time carnival funhouse.

Remember that there was always a part of the funhouse that was full of full-length sheets of clear glass? The route through the maze was quite confusing with all of its twists and turns. Just when you thought you knew which way to go, your nose would flatten against something hard and cold and the people outside who were watching would give a hoot and a holler as you stumbled back in surprise.

What was *your* strategy for successfully negotiating the hall of glass? Our technique was to cheat! If you looked down at the floor, you could usually see the thin line of molding that held the otherwise invisible panes of glass. As long as you didn't look up to see where you were going (and get distracted as a result), you could whiz through the maze with the speed of those eight-year-olds who were always running by everyone else while screaming at the top of their lungs. (They probably designed the maze to begin with!)

CHEAT? Who me? That's not fair! We know. It just happens to be the easiest way we know to teach someone how to challenge assumptions. When you get really good at challenging assumptions and you uncover a real doozy of a shared assumption, unconscious belief, or covert rule, people will say you are "cheating." (Even you may wonder about it!)

But this isn't a game, and your goal here is to come up with a new way of looking at things in order to resolve a difficulty. Kids change the rules to fit the players; you may be able to change the perspective to fit the problem.

We are *not* advocating that you cheat in earnest when playing with others. There are few ways we know that will spoil a good time quicker than that. We are simply suggesting that when all else fails to help you find an innovative solution to a persistent problem, you check to be sure you aren't being blinded by your own habits, expectations, and assumptions.

While you are at it, you might as well GENERATE ALTERNATIVES. Problem-solving is much more likely to be effective when you have lots of alternatives to consider. One creativity expert advocates that you look for the third "best" solution. That is, don't settle for the first one that shows up with good potential, keep on going until you have at least three "best solutions" to choose from.

With a little patience and some good hard playing

around with the possibilities (and impossibilities) you may arrive at an incredible treasure that otherwise would have remained hidden.

Be sure that what you are looking for doesn't always come in the *last* place you look. It makes sense on occasion to keep on looking even after you find what you think you want. It took Thomas Edison only about 1,000 attempts to whip out the electric light bulb.

If you haven't figured this out by now, in order to do all of these silly things, you will have to have perfected the ability to SUSPEND JUDGMENT—at least until you are ready to make good use of it. All too often we jump from inspiration to exasperation by evaluating critically whatever feeling, thought, or behavior dares to show its fragile beauty for more than a second. And we are just as hard on ourselves as we tend to be on others.

In this arena we can certainly learn from the wisdom of the young child. The Zen Buddhists have a saying that honors "beginner's mind," for in the mind of a beginner all things are possible, in the mind of the expert only a few.

Our willingness to explore options, play with possibilities, and avoid premature judgment are all elements of a more creative and rewarding work style. There *is* a time and place for evaluation and assessment; just make sure it doesn't eliminate the very solution it is intended to discover.

Activating your imagination, finding out what's good about it, using everything to your advantage, challenging assumptions, generating alternatives, and suspending judgment—all are marvelous ways of having fun while increasing your productivity. Just remember that the productivity in this case comes precisely from allowing yourself to have some space for fun-exploring possibilities first.

One new and exciting approach to incorporating the strategies listed above and building a sense of teamwork and cooperation among a group of co-workers at the same time is the use of ropes courses, "initiative" problems, or adventure games. These challenging activities combine the attractiveness of "play" with the riskiness of physically and mentally demanding problems to be solved.

With "chasms" to cross, "mountains" to climb, and "treasures" to find, active involvement is unavoidable. The heart pumps fast, the muscles tighten up, and the emotions run high when the group gets stuck and the problem seems unsolvable. But the cheers are real and the learning lasts when a solution is found.

For developing leadership, enhancing motivation, building self-confidence and team commitment, these action techniques are hard to beat. Sources for these activities can be found in the Resources section at the back of the book.

One final suggestion we have found helpful in increasing a sense of playfulness at work is to create your very own unique, portable, personalized *PLAYKIT* suitable for whatever work setting you inhabit.

If you are working an office job, for example, there are probably many times during the day when you are put on hold, the copier is stacked up, the computer goes down, or the boss wants to see you in "five minutes."

Any one of these interruptions can be irritating, frustrating, or at the very least boring as you wait them out. However, with your handy-dandy, do-it-yourself, low-cost Playkit, you can turn the situation to your advantage (got that?). The disruption becomes an excellent excuse to haul out a favorite "play-with" and start up your "Play Management Program" again.

You see, contrary to some bosses' opinions, neither the brain nor the body works very efficiently without periodic breaks in the action. Even when the change is simply to reach out to pick up your favorite "stroking stone," the result can be a decided decrease in detrimental stress. A momentary dose of enjoyment can unleash unexpected new energy. (And if you pick the right "play-withs," no one even needs to know you are busy enjoying your work!)

While your Playkit may look very different from ours, we will share some of our favorite items so that you can get the idea. The one I (Tobin) use most often is the familiar bright-red plastic egg filled with Silly Putty. The soothing yet stimulating motion of rolling, squeezing, stretching, and shaping the malleable stuff fills many a moment with a relaxing reminder of childhood days. And I can talk on the phone at the same time!

Then there is the collection of small but challenging puzzles—some filled with water, others with small steel balls that never go where you want them to—that I can draw on to refresh my mind and hands.

A small plastic box with brightly colored liquid that flows slowly down in intricate patterns is next to a magnetic paper-clip holder that calls on me to shape a new design in the air on a regular basis. A few smooth, polished stones are piled up next to a miniature sandscape that inverts at a flip of the wrist and creates an everchanging panorama of pleasing images.

Tom's counseling office is filled with attractively unique items that fairly beg to be handled. Small wax wizards compete for space with kaleidoscopes, puppets, and brilliantly reflective flat disks that glow with the colors of the rainbow as they spin. Then there are the trademark Vitamin C tablets in the shape of a heart that he has dubbed

Warm Fuzzies and that taste good, too. Many a youngster and middlester alike look forward to raiding the Warm Fuzzy jar.

The result of these few inexpensive items, available from any neighborhood gift store, is not a *dis*traction, but an *at*traction, a reminder that sitting at our desks, bench, or in our car can be something to look forward to and enjoy. They are our way of inviting the creativity of our Inner Child to grace the landscape of our adult lives.

You, too, can find your own "play-withs" that will be your anchor beyond "reality." Remember that assignment for regular trips to the toy store? Whether you need something portable, hideable, or shareable, if you will give yourself a few hours and a few bucks to shop with, you may recover some delightful treasures from your childhood that have remained hidden for years. It is all part of letting your child come out to play.

A fellow named Oswald B. Swallow summed up what we have been talking about here in the following eloquent and insightful verse:

CHOOSE TO HAVE FUN

Fun creates enjoyment
Enjoyment invites participation
Participation focuses attention
Attention expands awareness
Awareness promotes insight
Insight generates knowledge
Knowledge facilitates action
Action yields results.

Pleasure seems intimately tied to the paying of attention and the investment of energy. When we sense we are in control of our actions (or even act "as if" . . .) and the challenge is one we truly accept or choose, then the outcome can be merely a way to keep score; experiencing the "flow" itself becomes the real reward.

But don't just take our word for it. Turn to the next page and hear what some others have to say about play. Over the course of this book, we give you a range of opinion and insight from Plato to Pogo. And don't just take their word for it, either. Take a break—go out (or stay in) and play. Then, in the next part of this book, look at some possibilities for expanding your playgroup.

A Collection of Quotations (Part 1)

There is something in my stomach that knows everything. And that's what magic is.
CHRISTOPHER CORTHAY (AGE 6)

Among the many forms of life, man is the supreme player. Only man appears to play from birth to death . . . It seems the more advanced a species is on the evolutionary scale, the more frequent and diverse are its play activities.
EDWARD NORBECK

Whenever you trace the origin of a skill or practice which played a crucial role in the ascent of man, we usually reach the realm of play.
ERIC HOFFER

What seems to be the function of playfulness? The most general answer necessarily points to a quality of all things alive, namely the restoration and creation of a "leeway of mastery" in a set of developments or circumstances. . . . "free movement within prescribed limits."
ERIK ERIKSON

Children invite mystery, they invite opportunities for the incongruous, the unexplained, the half-revealed, the not knowing, the impending moment, the fear of the hidden, the tension of waiting, the anticipation of surprise, the possibility of danger, the savoring of darkness, the games of guessing, the condition of secrecy. And like explorers on a perilous cliff they lean over its edge looking for what will appear, hanging onto every surge of suspense, frozen in their gaze, as the unexpected slowly takes their breath away.

RICHARD LEWIS

Buffoonery is an essential element of good education. To be able to enjoy the unexpected, to perceive the incongruous, and to welcome the grotesque, is to start out with a good equipment to make sense of so strange a world as ours.

MARGARET LOWENFIELD

If you wish to glimpse inside a human soul and get to know a man, don't bother analyzing his ways of being silent, of talking, of weeping, or seeing how much he is moved by noble ideas; you'll get better results if you just watch him laugh. If he laughs well, he's a good man. . . .

DOSTOYEVSKI

"Believe me, my young friend, there is nothing —absolutely nothing—half so much worth doing as simply messing about in boats. Simply messing," he went on dreamily, "messing—about—in—boats; messing—"

"Look ahead, Rat!" cried the Mole suddenly.

It was too late. The boat struck the bank full tilt. The dreamer, the joyous oarsman, lay on his back at the bottom of the boat, his heels in the air.

"—about in boats—or with boats," the Rat went on composedly, picking himself up with a pleasant laugh. "In or out of 'em, it doesn't matter. Nothing seems really to matter, that's the charm of it. Whether you get away, or whether you don't; whether you arrive at your destination or whether you reach somewhere else, or whether you

never get anywhere at all, you're always busy, and you never do anything in particular and when you've done it there's always something else to do, and you can do it if you like, but you'd much better not."
  WATER RAT FROM *THE WIND IN THE WILLOWS,*
    BY KENNETH GRAHAME

Life is filled with insurmountable opportunities.
            POGO

Whatever else the child may suffer from, it does not suffer from remoteness of life, normally . . . it is fully alive, and that is why people, thinking back to their own childhood, long to have that naive vitality which they have lost in becoming grown-up. The child is an inner possibility, the possibility of renewal.
        MARIE LOUISE VON FRANZ

To be able to make-believe gives both the child and the adult a power over the environment and an opportunity to create one's own novelty and potential joy.
          DR. JEROME SINGER

The adult was once a child and a youth. He will never be either again: but neither will he ever be without the heritage of those former states. In fact, I would postulate that, in order to be truly adult, he must on each level renew some of the playfulness of childhood and some of the sportiveness of the young.
            ERIK ERIKSON

The only thing worth having in an earthly existence is a sense of humor.
          LINCOLN STEFFENS

PART
II

Building
Play Communities

8

The New Game Plan for Recovery

The Creator made man able to do everything—talk, run, look, and hear. He was not satisfied, though, till man could do just one thing more—and that was: LAUGH. And so man laughed and laughed and laughed. And the Creator said: "Now you are fit to live."
APACHE INDIAN MYTH

Hello, I'm Tobin Quereau . . . And I'm Tom Zimmermann . . . and we're here to welcome you to The New Game Plan for Recovery, a program we designed for use at conferences, in treatment centers, for weekend workshops and such—anywhere people gather who would like to bring more play into their day and more life into their lives. . . .

And so it begins. Sometimes for two hours, sometimes four, sometimes for a whole day or more. In cafeterias and classrooms, banquet halls and boardrooms, parks and playgrounds. For groups of ten, fifty, five hundred and more. We have been giving this workshop since 1982 in various forms and locations across the country, and we have *finally* gotten it into print.

For all those of you who have played with us over the years (and who have inquired about, asked for, demanded, and insisted that we write this all down) we are eternally grateful. Our lives have been enriched by your trust, courage, enthusiasm, joy, delight, and playfulness. In truth, we could not do this without *you*!

What follows is our best try at approximating what we do when we present The New Game Plan for Recovery to people in the field of chemical dependency. With modifications we have also found it appropriate for the general areas of stress management, team-building, communication skills, classroom management, and family, organizational, and community development. It changes somewhat every time we do it, but there are certain elements and activities we just can't seem to leave out, so over the years it has become a part of us—just as the people we present it to do.

Our debt is great to the people who began the "New Games" movement in the early 1970s. Before we met, both of us had the privilege to be trained by people from the New Games Foundation. Their books (*New Games*, and *More New Games*) and their work (or rather, play) confirmed for us the possibility that there were others out there in the world who valued cooperative play, fun, and humor in much the way we did. Many of the activities we use as a basis for The New Game Plan we learned from those New Games folks, and we thank them wherever they are.

While we are at it, we also thank Matt Weinstein and Joel Goodman for their influence on us. Their work through the *Playfair* book and organization and through the Humor Project continue to be a model for what we are about. Many of the exercises we present we have stolen from these two guys. If you ever get the chance to play with either of them, don't pass it up, and say hello to them for us.

In the tradition of these master players we encourage you to make the most of your playful side and share what you learn here with others. The games we learned, the ones we made up, and the ones we have yet to learn from you are all part of the universal and never-ending tradition of people at play. They belong to none of us and to all of us. Pass 'em on.

Now back to the workshop. Enjoy!

We developed this material not to deal with the "miserable drunk," but to prevent the "miserable sober." It is designed to counteract the "isms," alcoholism, workaholism, even criticism! (We wanted to have something in here for everyone.) It can work well for chemical dependency, co-dependency, and independency—those are the ones of us who just think we haven't been affected by drugs and alcohol in our lives.

As part of our program we plan on breaking some rules— particularly the rules of chemically dependent, dysfunctional families: Don't talk. Don't trust. Don't feel. By the time we finish we will have you talking, trusting, and feeling—and feeling really good. That's because we have found that when people feel good, they begin to feel good, and feelings are at the heart of recovery from this family disease.

Along the way we hope you'll recover your sense of hope, your sense of joy, and your sense of humor. You see, chemicals are mood-altering substances . . . and so are we! We just go about it in a more naturally satisfying way. But we will need your help. Are you willing to help us? (scattered cheers) ARE YOU WILLING TO HELP US?? (SHOUTS, WHISTLES, AND APPLAUSE) All right! Let's start by breaking some rules.

What should we do first, Tom?

How about that rule that you should never talk to strangers?

O.K., let's see, will all the strangers please raise their hands. . . .

We hope you are beginning to get the idea. We move fairly quickly into involving the audience in what we are doing. The first series of exercises we call *Ice Melters*. Beginning with *Kicking Out the Strangers*, they go something like this . . .

Kicking Out the Strangers

All right, you said you would help us. Strangers can be friends we just haven't met yet. And we know now that we can't do this alone, so your job is to stand up, look around you and introduce everyone you see to everyone else. And we only have about fifty-two and a half seconds allocated for this exercise, so get to it!

The general melee of sound and movement is enough to destroy any sense of propriety and decorum in even those struggling hardest to maintain them. Their only out lies in the fact that during this exercise no one really pays attention to anyone else for much longer than five seconds anyway.

After a suitable time (we never remember to measure it), we whistle and stomp and wave until we get their attention back, and from that moment on we (and they) are on our way.

We have found it particularly effective to follow the introductions exercise with one we call *Saying Good-bye*. We set it up this way:

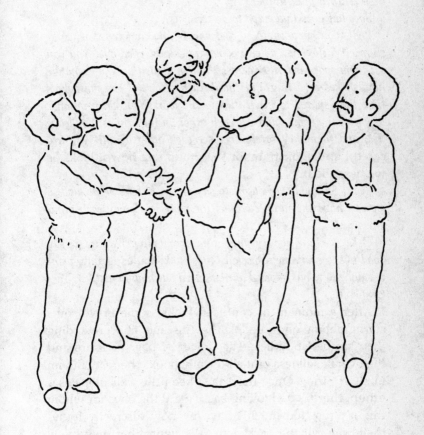

Kicking Out the Strangers

Saying Good-bye

You know, Tobin, that reminds me of a rule my mother always told me. "Save the best for last." A corollary was, "Don't eat dessert until after dinner."

So what does that have to do with us?

Well, you know the very best part of any conference or workshop? It's the end, when people are saying good-bye. You can see them spot each other across the room, rush up and exchange handshakes or a hug and thank each other for the marvelous time they shared together during the workshop. They promise to write, they smile and pat each other on the arm as they leave . . . and then they rarely ever see each other again! (We are careful to demonstrate for the group just how it looks as we describe it.)

Yeah! So maybe we ought to say our good-byes right now so we can have the next few days (or hours) to enjoy each other afterward!

O.K., we have about eighty-nine seconds to make sure we say good-bye to everyone, especially those folks you especially want to say hello to but haven't quite figured out how to just yet. . . . Go for it!

After a moment of confused looks, some brave souls start grabbing on to people they just met and pretending they are best buddies. The power of peer pressure and the overall silliness of it all usually hooks the rest of them in short order. Once they have been this ridiculous as a group, there is no looking back. (And the ones for whom this is "just too much" have by now discreetly found their way out the back door. We figure that they know what they can and can't handle, and maybe they will stick around longer next time.)

Along about this point in the presentation we have to haul out our collection of train whistles, sirens, and general noisemakers, since the room is by now in a fairly disrupted state. We may stand on chairs if we

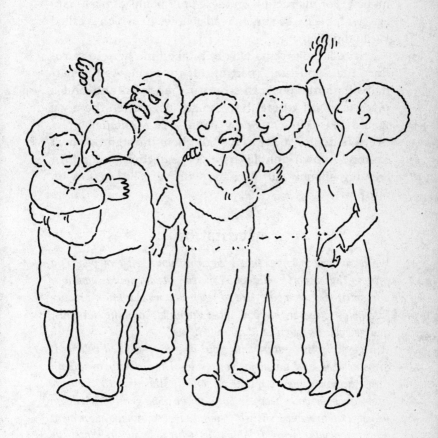

Saying Good-bye

aren't already up on a stage in order to get people's attention.

Part of keeping The New Game Plan working is carefully assessing when to interrupt what we have set in motion. For instruction on these finer points of play management, please be sure to read chapter 10, which is called Facilitating Fun.

Before large groups we often take time here to introduce the ''spiritual'' part of our program. As the participants sort themselves out of the crowd and find a place to stand where they can see us, we tell them we would like them to know about our *Meditation* practice. We demonstrate as we talk them through this next exercise (which doubles as a very effective method for creating silence out of chaos with very little effort on our part).

Meditation

We want you to know that recovering your sense of play is a process that involves the whole person—body, mind, emotion, and spirit. So we would like to teach you a meditation practice that helps to center the body, quiet the mind, calm the emotions, and get you in touch with your ''higher'' self.

It goes like this—start with your body straight and balanced, arms relaxed and down by your side. Then slowly raise both arms, keeping them straight as you lift them, until they are high up above your head. Finally, lower them gently back down as you exhale a soft ''shshsh'' sound. The sound and movement stop when your arms are down by your side again. Watch us once and then we will do it together.

Once we take the group through the exercise, a profound stillness spreads through the room. We then let them know that whenever they see either of us standing up at the front of the room with our hands over our heads going ''shhh!'' they should stop whatever they are do-

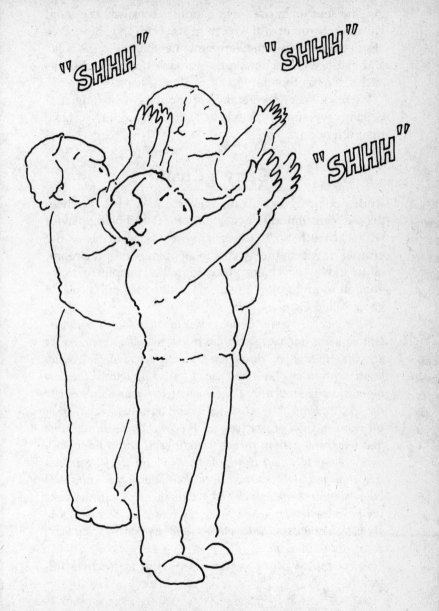

Meditation

ing and join us in the "meditation." That way the room will soon be quiet and we can get on with the show. (We also let them know they are now members of our "cult" and can leave any donations, valuables, or Rolls Royces at the door as they leave.)

It works! When we get tired of shouting, whistling, and waving, we simply "meditate" sibilantly until we have their attention.

Carry a Chair

At this point we usually do a few more *Ice Melters* to help people feel comfortable making contact and being playful with each other. At times it is necessary to move the group away from their chairs to an open part of the room, or to move the chairs away from the people to make enough room to play. In such situations we might play a game called *Carry a Chair*.

All right everybody, we want you to know that it is important to warm up adequately when you intend to play, so we are going to take you through a few exercises to loosen you up before continuing. Let's all raise our arms up toward the ceiling again and stretch up tall. Now stretch your hands out to the left, and to the right. Now reach down and grab hold of the chair in front of you (you see the benefits of sitting in the first row?) and with your back straight gently lift it up slightly off the floor. Now put it back down. Now lift it up again and this time put it back down over there along the wall. And when you finish come back and get another one until we have the room cleared for action so we can continue. Be sure not to stumble over purses, water glasses, and notebooks as you make your way to the wall.

A couple of other variations on the *Ice Melters* follow.

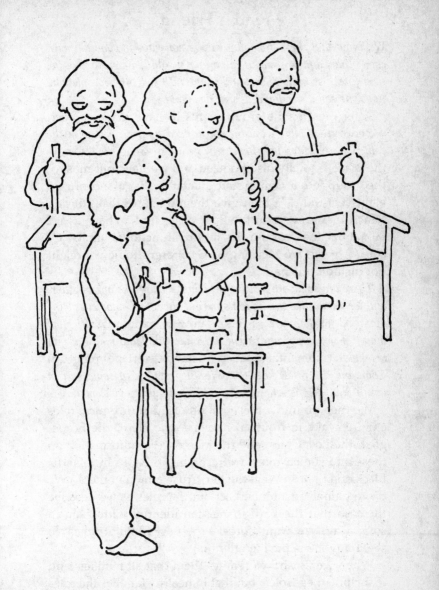

Carry a Chair

Find a Friend

We know that there are many things you have in common with each other, and to prove it to you we would like you to take the next fifteen seconds to find and stand with two other people who have the same size hand as you do. Go!

After most of the group seems to have made contact, we continue: *Now we want you to find someone else with the same color eyes as you have.* As you can imagine, by now the place is totally disorganized and we have put most of the group into a mental state similar to that of a confused eight-year-old. We then give them a short break (during which they can sit on the floor or go find a chair) as we talk about the typical roles in a dysfunctional family. Of course, if we are focusing on a different topic we might not include this part.

There are some other ways in which we are like one another, and we would like to talk to you about them for a moment. How many of you here are parents? (show of hands) *Great! How many of you are grandparents? Wonderful! How many of you are kids?* (momentary pause as hands start popping up) *Come on, we're all kids too! We all grew up in some sort of family and that is what we would like to talk to you about.*

We then go into a presentation of the four typical roles children take in troubled families—the Hero, the Scapegoat, the Lost Child, and the Mascot. (For information on these and similar roles, we recommend books by Claudia Black and Sharon Wegscheider-Cruse, among others.) We try to ham it up a bit and act out the roles as we describe them so that the participants can identify with them in some way. We even "forget" the Lost Child at times, to see if anyone is paying attention.

When we finish, we remind them that all families tend to include these roles, but that in healthy families the roles are not as limiting, rigid, or intense as they can be in troubled families. We then ask the participants to decide

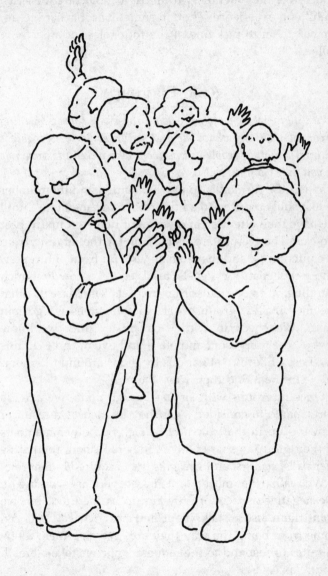

Find a Friend

which role they identify with most as reflecting their *own* childhood experience. Though sometimes it is hard to do, we ask them to pick one of the four roles for an activity called—

Role Playing

As a way to get to know more about those you share something in common with, you have the next sixty seconds to get together with all *the other people in this room who picked the same role as you did. Go find 'em!*

When the turmoil is somewhat settled and the number of lost souls reduced to a minimum, we "meditate" until we have their attention and we identify the groups as best we can. The Heroes are usually by far the largest group at conferences, and they usually end up front and center. The Scapegoats or Rebels tend to be a rowdy bunch standing off to one side or in the back. The Mascots often are the smallest group of all, so sometimes we go join them. We check in with each cluster until we know "who" they represent and often find two or three clumps of "Lost Children" at various locations around the room. We help them find their way "home."

Once in groups with similar backgrounds, we ask the participants to consider what they learned as a result of growing up in that role and to pick two other members of their group to share with as they talk about the particular *skills*, *abilities*, and *strengths* they acquired in that role.

We realize that most people in recovery are working on the negative aspects of growing up as they did, but we want them also to talk about and hear what *benefits* can come from being the way they are. We give them a few minutes to respond to the request while we take a breath and relax. . . .

When we are ready to go again (just *before* people seem to be running out of what they have to say) we introduce

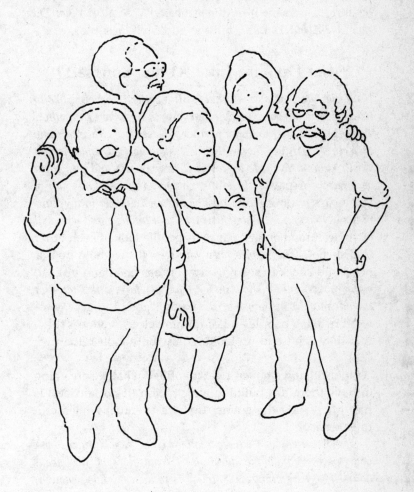

Role Playing

one of our all-time favorite exercises. This one works with any group—post office employees, principals, real estate salespeople, teachers, hospital workers, you name it! Just be sure to present it enthusiastically! We call it *What Do You Like About Yourself*, but we don't tell *them* that. . . .

What Do You Like About Yourself?

Now that you know each other a little better, we would like to help you find out some really interesting things about each other. To begin, you need to find a partner. Please raise either a thumb or a finger. (Index *finger, Rebels!*) *Now go find someone you* don't *know who made the same choice you did and pick them as a partner.* (pause) *Just one partner.* (pause) *O.K., all of you groups of three please raise your hand and get into groups of two! Now decide in your pair who will be apple and who will be orange.* (momentary pause as people look at each other in disbelief) *Fine, apples raise your stem* (as we hold up our hand and check to see if every pair has one hand up). *All right, now oranges, show us your navel! No—wait! That's for the advanced workshop. Sorry.* (Humor goes a long way toward relaxing people and, if nothing else, convinces them that they can't end up looking any more foolish than we do.)

Notice that we haven't yet identified what we are going to have them do. Building anticipation (if not anxiety) is part of creating the energy that we eventually release in the exercise.

O.K., now apples we have a job for you. We want you to ask your partner a simple question. "What do you like about yourself?" And oranges, your job is to answer. Easy enough, isn't it.

Here we throw in an additional exercise if we have the time. It heightens the energy level and prolongs the suspense of *What Do You Like About Yourself*. It is called . . .

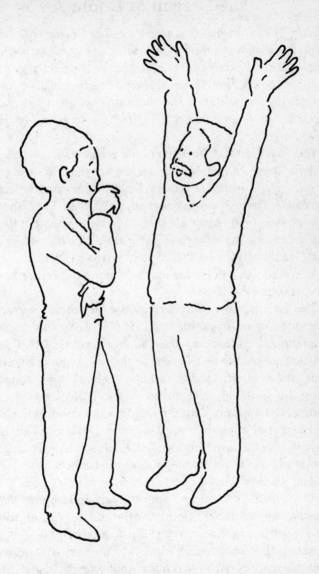

What Do You Like About Yourself?

The Dragon of Doubt

Hold it, Tom. I'm afraid it's here again. The Dragon of Doubt. I saw it slip into the room as you said "like about yourself." People started looking anxious, the hair on their necks started to rise. I can see it up there, clinging on their shoulders, hissing into their ears, "There ain't nothing good about you, turkey!" Before we go on we're going to have to get rid of that thing for good.

Yeah, I can smell it from here. Let's get after it.

Before we go on with the exercise, we are going to show you how to get rid of the Dragon of Doubt lurking in your consciousness. First put one foot in front of the other. Then stretch your arms in front of you like this. Now, on the count of three pull your elbows back hard as you shout "HUNH!" and knock that Dragon off your back! One, two, three—HUNH!

NO, NO, don't tickle the dragon! Do it all together now. One, two, three—HUNH!

This isn't working. That Dragon has been there for years. You have to give it your all to get rid of it. Look, let's try one more thing. This time let's shout all together, "GET OFF MY BACK!" as you jab that Dragon in the ribs, knock it onto the floor, and stomp it into the ground! And don't forget to wipe any extra scales off your partner's back. (All of this is, of course, dynamically demonstrated for the unbelieving audience.) *And remember, the Dragon of Doubt can look like anyone—I mean anything, so just think of whatever dragon you would like to get rid of—no one ever needs to know what or who you have in mind. Ready, set, GO! "GET . . . OFF . . . MY . . . BACK!"* (stomp, pound, slap and shout) *Now, doesn't that feel better?* (loud cheers and applause) *Yeah! And if you can be that silly, you can do anything!*

Now back to our exercise, apples, for the next sixty seconds you ask oranges, "What do you like about yourself?", and when they answer, you nod, say that's great and then you ask, "What else do you like about yourself?"

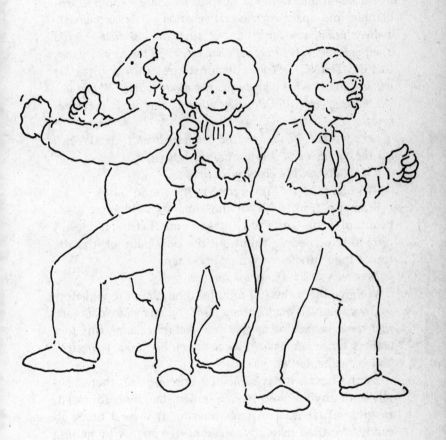

The Dragon of Doubt

Wait a minute, Tom. You forgot something. What about brain freeze?

You would *think of that, Tobin. All right, for* some *of you there may be a temporary phenomenon called brain freeze. Tobin will demonstrate.* (After a suspicious glare, Tobin stares blankly into space for several seconds.) *If, due to anxiety and confusion, you can't think of anything* else *that you like about yourself, just throw both hands high in the air and shout, ''EVERYTHING!''* (Tobin demonstrates) *Then your partner will ask you, ''What* else *do you like about yourself?'' and you will have to come up with some other answer or get very tired arms.*

Let's practice. You all pretend you have brain freeze. We will ask the question and you practice the response.

''What do you like about yourself?''

''EVERYTHING!'' (everyone in the room)

From up front with all those hands held high it's a beautiful sight—and even if it isn't entirely true, it doesn't hurt to have people shout out the possibility of it at the top of their lungs every now and then.

Now let's do it. Apples ask oranges, go!

We give them the full minute, then blow the whistles.

Great. You did fine! Nobody died? You did so well, in fact, that we have decided to give you another chance. This time oranges get to ask apples ''What do you like about yourself?'' You know the routine, go!

By the time we have finished this exercise, there usually isn't anyone who hasn't smiled, laughed, chuckled, or grinned (at least in embarrassment) several times already. We then take advantage of this energy by getting people together in small-group work. As you read through these exercises, you may spot the pattern of group building we initiate. From relating to one other person, we build to a group of four, then eight, and so on. Depending on the size of the audience, we may carry

this on for several repetitions to bring eventually everyone together again in the end.

It is all part of the process of making strangers into
friends we *have* met!

Introduce Glowingly

*Fantastic! You have now broken one of society's dumbest rules—
don't speak highly of yourself. Some people go so far as to not
even think highly of themselves. That kind of attitude is not
good for anyone. Practice thinking and speaking highly of yourself whenever possible.*

*And just so we balance the process out fairly, we also want
you to practice speaking highly of someone else! You now know
several fascinating and valuable things about your partner. You
do remember those things they told you, don't you?*

*We would like you now to take your partner, find a pair to
join up with so you are in groups of four, and introduce your
partner to the other two people GLOWINGLY! If you experience
a brief bout of brain freeze, fake it till you make it. . . . Hit it!*

In the ensuing chaos of *Introduce Glowingly*, we invariably see people who didn't know each other ten
minutes previously standing together holding hands or
patting each other on the back and, sure enough, practically glowing with positive feelings. That plus tons of
shared laughter.

We continue to build on this growing bond by asking
the groups of four to join with one another to make
groups of eight. Here, to make sure no one thinks we are
just full of fun and games, we introduce a problem called
Knots.

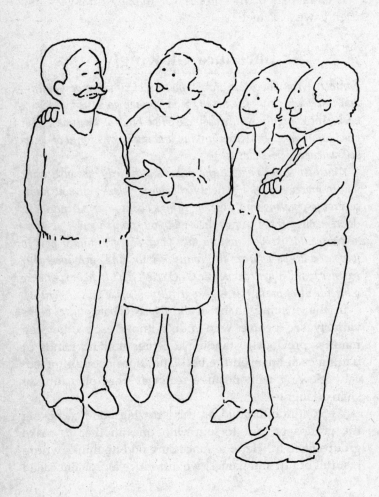

Introduce Glowingly

Knots

(Shhh-ing them into silence) *All right, you are now in groups of eight. We are about to teach you some problem-solving techniques. Anyone here have a problem?* (only a few hands go up) *See, Tobin, I told you we were working with denial . . . Anyone here* not *have any problems?* (more honesty emerges spontaneously) *Anyway, pay attention, because if you don't have any problems yet, we are going to give you one.*

But first we want to teach you the three C's of problem solving. Number one is Communicate. That means be sure to listen as much as you speak. Number two is Cooperate. You can't solve this problem alone. Number three is Create. This problem may be unlike any you have ever had before, so you will need to be creative.

Stand in your circle, shoulder to shoulder, and reach across the circle to take the hand of someone on the other side. Don't let go. Now reach across with your other hand and take the hand of someone else! Be sure you do not *have the hand of the person on either side of you and that you do have the hands of two different people across the circle.*

You now have a knot, and the problem will be to work together to untangle your knot without letting go until you are in a nice big round circle. It can be done! (Sometimes.) Just be sure not to break any bones along the way.

We usually wander through the room to assess the progress and frustration and occasionally to kibitz. When most of the groups that have any hope of succeeding have made it, usually with loud shrieks and clapping when they do, we get the participants' attention and do some more "teaching."

Let's give everyone a big hand. You did wonderfully, even those of you back in the corner who are still struggling to untie the untieable knot and who are not yet paying attention to us. You see, we forgot to present to you the fourth "C" of problem solving—when all else fails, Cheat!

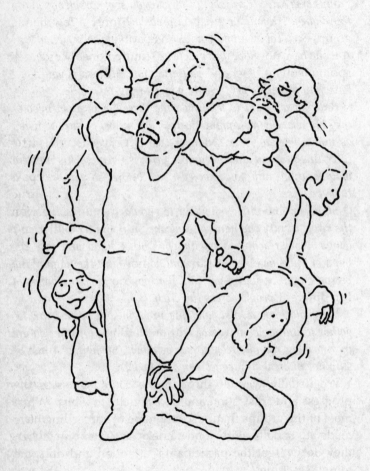

Knots

Actually, the fact is that sometimes despite our grandest efforts and noblest intentions, things don't turn out the way we want them to. In such cases one may want to consider the wisdom of learning to let go. *It is a practice we can all benefit from. . . .*

We also noticed a few of the folks stuck in the smack-dab middle of their knot who looked suspiciously like they were enjoying their problem! Those are the ones to look out for. . . .

For the next activity we stay in our group of eight. We give our groups a chance to feel what it is like to really be supported by a group of friends. We call this one *Support Circle* or *Willows in the Wind*. Since it is one of the most powerful exercises for evoking the experience of once again becoming like a child, we take careful steps to insure it is a positive one. We are specific with the instructions, and usually one of us moves through the room making sure things are going smoothly as the other one handles the changes from up front.

Willows in the Wind

Stay in your circles of eight and we will do a different sort of activity to help you feel just what it is to be supported in what you do. We need one brave person to step to the center of your circle and stand with his or her feet together, arms crossed over his or her chest. The rest of the group stands around the outside with one foot forward, one foot back, and hands raised in front of their chest, palms forward toward the person in the center.

The one in the center is going to close his or her eyes, keeping his or her body straight like a willow tree, as he or she begins to lean in any direction until the people on the outside catch him or her gently with their hands and pass them slowly around the circle. It helps if the people on the outside softly whistle like the wind as they move the person around the circle. This is a trust *exercise, and we want you to treat*

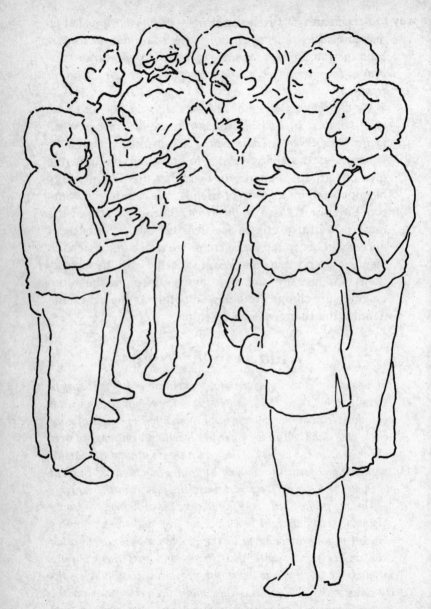

Willows in the Wind

each other as you would like to be treated. Stay close together and work as a team. Remember, slowly and gently. . . .

For this one, we always have playing in the background some soothing music featuring sounds in Nature, and one of us moves constantly about the room to insure that people are following the rules and acting safely. We particularly want to avoid having a group get rowdy and disruptive as a way of dealing with uncomfortable feelings.

One of us gives the directions to change the person in the center every couple of minutes until everyone has had a chance to volunteer. We make sure no one is forced into moving into the middle. We have been known in such cases to ask a reluctant participant if we might take his or her place for a turn. He or she is generally relieved and we are always delighted for the chance to get the support!

This exercise is a powerful one. Sometimes it brings on tears, and we generally give people some time afterward to talk to each other about what they found felt best and what was toughest. This can be a very intimate time for the groups, and we want them to have space to absorb the experience.

After slowing down the pace with this exercise, we generally crank things up again afterward with a game called *Instant Replay*.

Instant Replay

Can we have your attention, please? Now that you have shared some time with members of your group, we want you to get to know some more friends that you didn't know you had. Each group of eight join with another group of eight to make a group of sixteen. This next game will help you to learn the names of all of the rest of the members of your group.

How many of you have ever seen a TV? You have? O.K., then how many of you have ever seen an instant replay? Wow!

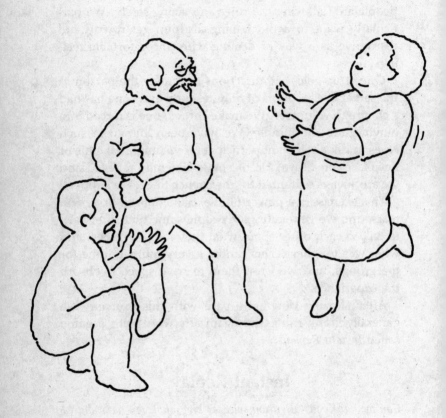

Instant Replay

Maybe they know this game, Tom. At any rate, we are going to have you be the instant replay camera for a very special game. Starting with the tallest member of your circle—you are in a circle, aren't you?—each of you will have a chance to jump to the middle of the circle one at a time, shout out your name, and pantomime a favorite thing you do for fun. It looks something like this . . . (one of us demonstrates).

As soon as you finish acting out your chosen activity you leap back out of the middle of the circle and the rest of the group becomes the replay camera. They jump all together into the middle just like you did, shout out your name, and do an exact copy of what you did a moment before. You stay where you are and enjoy the show!

When they jump back it is the next person's turn. Continue until everyone around the circle has had a chance to share one of their favorite pastimes. You are on your own. Go!

By now things look like they are a real mess—people shouting at the top of their lungs, "dancing" around the room, swinging "golf clubs," "skiing," "gardening," "bicycling," and occasionally "meditating" in the headstand position! (That one rarely receives a total "replay.") But there is method to the madness, and eventually all of the groups come to a stop, panting and clapping in delight that they made it through without forgetting their own name. Of course no one remembers anyone else's, but then we really didn't expect them to. . . .

Carrying this energy one more step, we then move into *People to People*. If the group is of manageable size, say 150 or less, we make one or two large groups for this one, with one of us in charge of each group. If we have more than that, we might blend four groups of sixteen together to make several circles of sixty-four and just lead them all from up front.

People to People

For this next exercise everyone needs a partner and one person stands alone in the center (generally one of us, to start with). This is a simple activity to help you get in touch with your partner. The person in the center begins by calling out a set of body parts like this—"hand to hand." Everyone in the circle then puts their hands up to the hands of their partner and we are on our way. The "caller" continues two or three more times with different body parts—head to head, back to back—as the group follows their instructions.

Finally, after getting tired of watching the others have all the fun, the caller yells out "PEOPLE TO PEOPLE!" At this point everyone has to leave their place and go find another partner (especially the caller) and the person who ends up without a partner is the "winner" and gets to be the next caller!

(Sometimes in the confusion the original caller ends up without a partner and has to lead the next round. Watch out! That person will tend to be more vicious the second time around—head to foot, knee to back—any torturous position.)

It helps if we can get a little rhythm going as we call out, so everyone snap their fingers—A-one, and two, and three, and— EAR TO EAR!

For very experienced groups of quick learners, we may prescribe a round of *"Cumulative People to People."* In this case, everyone has to hold each position while adding the next one to it. In the hands of an out of touch (or vicious) caller, this one can become a chiropractor's nightmare . . . and loads of fun!

After several people have had a turn as caller and several others have been snatched nearly limb from limb by competing partner-hunters in full panic, we call out "New Game!" and gather the whole group into one large circle for

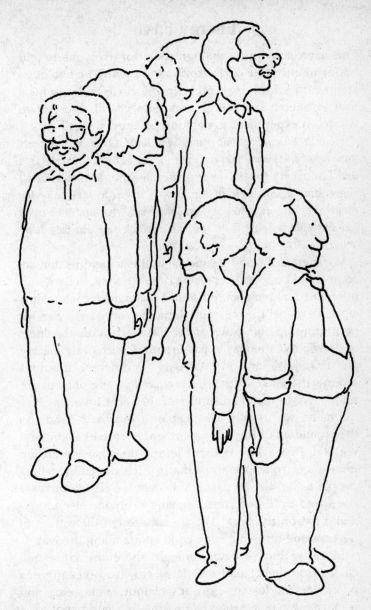

People to People

Energy Pass

This exercise requires enough room for everyone to join hands in one large circle around the room. The two of us stand across from each other in the circle and talk for a moment about the energy that connects all of us. Then we do an experiment to demonstrate how it works.

Now that we are in one group, you have a chance to connect with all of the people you have seen here, but not yet met. Tom and I are going to send some of the energy of love that we all share around the circle in the form of a gentle squeeze of the hand. Pay attention to your next-door neighbor and when you feel the squeeze, pass it on. Let's see which side can pass it on faster.

We then each send a squeeze in the same direction accompanied by sounds of racing cars, whoops, hollers, and other encouragements. It doesn't really matter who wins, since we all get the message along the way—but when we each jump up and down as the jolt reaches us, the effect is electric. We then try to pass a sound, each of us starting an "OOOOW" and an "AAAAH" in different directions around the circle. It gets pretty hairy as the ones in the middle try to pass and receive at the same time.

Finally, we usually ask people to put their hands on the shoulders of the persons on either side of them, and we play *Pass a Pat*. Without letting on what we are up to, we start one pat at a time in each direction, telling people to be sure to pass it on, then we slowly increase the speed until everyone is giving everyone else an ongoing pat on the back. We are sure to tell them they all deserve one for being such good sports along the way.

Since we have by now brought the entire group full circle—from being part of a large crowd to meeting one other person, to pairs, groups of four, eight, etc., and back to the whole group again—this is a good spot for a break. This part of the New Game Plan for Recovery takes

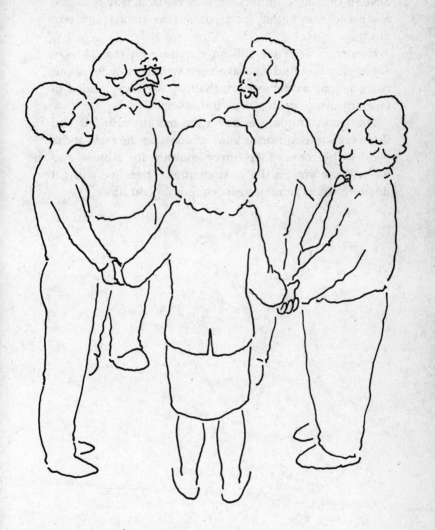

Energy Pass

about an hour and a half; and if that is all the time we have, it can stand on its own as a valuable way to create a sense of community and connection among any size group.

However, since we still have quite a bit more to say about play and find we have been writing now for about twice as long as the average chapter, we have decided to take advantage of the break ourselves.

The water fountain is down the hall on your left and there are some soft drinks and goodies on the table at the back of the room. Take fifteen minutes for a break and we will see you in the next chapter. There we will get down to some genuine, get 'em goin' good times.

9

The New Game Plan in Action

Why do we create games that give us purpose only so we can, by playing them well together, be released from all purpose?

It is a balancing act. It is a dialog—a play between. On the one hand there is silliness, on the other seriousness. On this side confusion, on this clarity. Here delight, here despair. It is neither work nor play, purpose nor purposelessness that satisfies us. It is the dance between.

BERNARD DE KOVEN

When we come back from the break, we usually want to liven things up, so we might start with a game we call the fastest game in the world. That gets people's attention and distracts them from the real title, which is *Everybody's It!* Come in a little closer and we will tell you how it goes. . . .

Everybody's It

Welcome back! Everyone come on in close now so we can tell you about this next game, which happens to be the fastest game in the world. Want to see it again? Nahh, we're kidding about that, we haven't played it yet. But if you will all gather around us so we don't have to shout, we will tell you how to play Everybody's It. *Come on up close, pretend you are among friends!*

Anyone ever play freeze tag? O.K., this is just like that with a special twist. If you tag someone, they are frozen. If someone tags you, you are frozen. Got it? The only other thing you have to remember is the name of the game, which is . . . EVERY-BODY'S IT!

At this point some folks get the idea and start tagging like mad anyone they can reach. Most people though stand in confusion until they are frozen on the spot, and a few sly dogs slip to the outside of the crowd and run like crazy around the room to avoid getting frozen. Since we pulled everyone in tight, usually the action is over in about five to seven seconds for most of the group (us included) and we then decisively declare the game over and single out some successful, slippery soul as the winner. If the group seems to be up for it, we might go on to play a variation of the game called *Everybody's It Wounded Tag*. (How's that for a dumb name?)

In this game the first time you get tagged, you have just been wounded and need to put one hand over the place you were tagged in order to protect the wound. You are still mobile, however, and capable of tagging others as long as you keep the wound covered. After a second tag (not on the foot, we hope!) you use your other hand to cover that wound and you move as quickly as you can to stay out of anyone else's reach. (Gentle "butt" tags on others are still permissible, but not kicks or body blocks.)

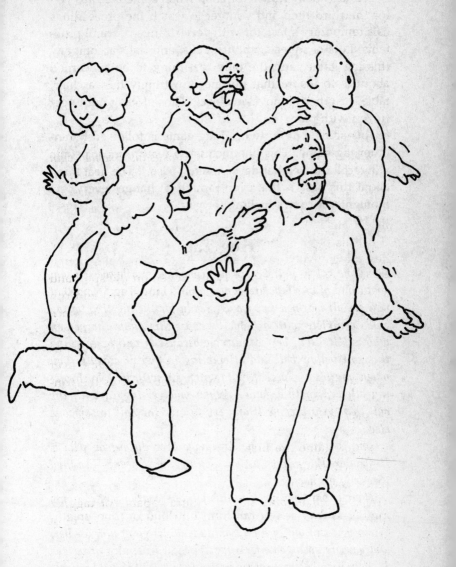

Everybody's It

You are finally frozen for good when someone zaps you for the third time and you get to watch the proceedings as a temporary spectator with very strange postural problems. Lots of squeals, shouts, eeks, and hahs accompany this tag game, and the only real thing to be concerned about is to insure that no one unwittingly tags a chair, table, or other immovable object. Those folks tend to get frozen with pain.

This active but fairly brief tag game is followed by another tag game. This one includes a feature most people will recall from earlier days—a safe "base." The neat thing about this base is that even though it changes every few moments, it comes looking for you!

Hug Tag

Everyone catch your breath for a moment while we tell you about one of our favorite games of all, Hug Tag. *Now that you are all warmed up, we are ready for the big time, a tag game complete with a home base. In this game the person who is "It" will be recognizable because It will be carrying this soft yellow ball and attempting to give it away to you when you least expect it by tagging you with it. (No throwing allowed in this game.) When you get tagged with the ball then you become It and try to give the ball to someone else.*

You, however, have one advantage over the person who is It—you are safe as long as you are hugging someone—like this! (See why we like it?)

There is only one catch to this lovely scenario, you can only hug for as long as you can hum out loud on one breath. When you run out of hum, you have to let go of him (or her) and you are open game for a tag. Tired or frustrated or vicious Its have been known to stand patiently by with the ball hovering over someone's head as they hummed their swan song.

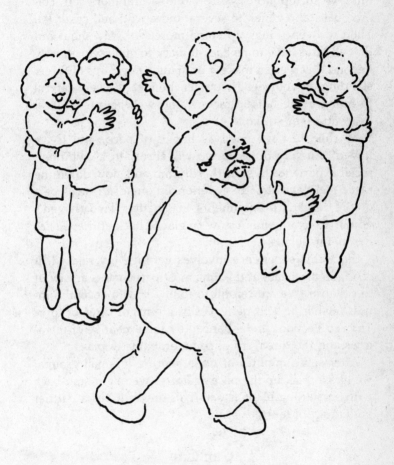

Hug Tag

Any hug in a storm will do, just make sure for now that it's only for two! Here I come!

This game goes on with one It for about two minutes until we surreptitiously throw out several more soft, colored balls and generate several more wild and crazy Its. Then to liven things up some more, we may shout out that all hugs have to be back-to-back to qualify for safety. Beyond that we can make it only hugs in groups of three, standing on your head, you get the idea. Be very careful to monitor the fatigue factor, stop well before the first heart attack or stroke.

By this time we need a change of pace, and if we haven't already done so we will throw in a childhood recall experience to shift the rhythm and slow down the race. You have already experienced one of these as part of the research assignments in Chapter Two (haven't you?). Take a moment now to glance back at the *Guided Replay* for details.

Since this experience involves getting very relaxed, it can fit in nicely about the time most participants are about to collapse. We are careful to follow it with several minutes of sharing of experiences in groups of three or four. The recollections are enhanced by the exchange of memories and the discovery of common paths to play.

After some minutes of open sharing in small groups, we like to pick up the pace again, so we might start back with something like *Car Car*. This one requires a partner and an act of faith.

Car Car

Now that we have started remembering some of our childhood pleasures, let's try one of them on. Everyone find a partner of approximately the same height, if possible. Decide who is going to go first. (Leave a little suspense in the air by not speci-

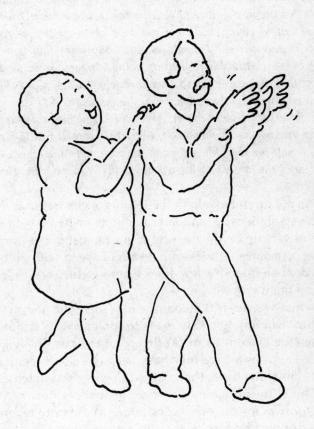

Car Car

fying why—those who go first will feel braver and those who decline will feel smarter!)

Now the one who is going first please put up your bumpers so we can play Car Car. *Put your hands up in front of your body, palms forward, arms bent to absorb any unexpected contact. You are now a car and your partner is the driver. Drivers stand behind your vehicle and put your hands on the steering wheel—your partner's shoulders. It is important that you be able to see clearly where you are going, drivers, since we all know that cars can't see to drive themselves. Cars, please close your eyes now and learn what it really means to TRUST!*

Drivers, start your engines. We will begin with a leisurely drive around the neighborhood, being very careful not to have any fender benders. Move around the room with the other cars and enjoy the lovely weather we are having. You too, cars. Have fun!

We are careful to add in the sounds of city traffic as the trip gets underway, and after a minute or two we direct the drivers up on the freeway so we can get out of town. That, of course, entails an increase of speed with an occasional siren and a few honks from eighteen-wheelers along the way.

When we reach the countryside, there are the mandatory winding two-lane roads to contend with until we reach the lookout point. At this point the cars finally get to look out on where they have been (we don't mention the numerous times they peeked in sheer self-defense).

The virtues of going first become evident next as we *switch roles* for the drive back home! We simply reverse the scenery and pace for the return trip, and those drivers who were reckless on the way out tend to find out what it feels like to be driven crazy on the way back in.

If you have never really tried this at "freeway speeds," be sure to do so yourself *prior* to suggesting it to others. The thrill of being "blacked out" can easily turn into the panic of being bashed into, so firsthand experience is essential for a front-line facilitator interested in keeping things fun.

In preparation for another exercise, we need to divide the group into three roughly equal parts. *Psychic Shake* is a playful way to accomplish that task.

Psychic Shake

Already tonight, we have found many ways in which we are like one another—but we want you to realize how connected we really can be. How many of you are psychic? (Usually we get a couple of hands) *Well, even though you might not realize it, we are all psychic in some way or another and this next game is going to prove it.*

Each of us has a favorite number—1, 2, or 3. (If you didn't know that, you do now.) Tom and I will demonstrate how to determine psychically if another person shares that same number as his or her favorite. Observe.

Here Tom and I approach each other and after a brief pause to "communicate" our special number silently, we reach out and shake hands in an exaggerated fashion, pumping our hands once, twice, or three times to indicate the number we had chosen. If we are "on," both of us stop moving at the same time. If not, one of us ends up yanking up when the other is stopping and the error is clearly evident. Most of the time we are "on," but it is more fun when we aren't.

Now it is your turn. Choose your favorite number—1, 2, or 3—and move around the room until you collect all the other people who have chosen the same number as you. Remember, no talking. This is your chance to see how well you can "sense" who your soul mates are.

After another bout of confused milling around, three generally distinct groups of people begin to emerge. We check to make sure that all of the group members agree

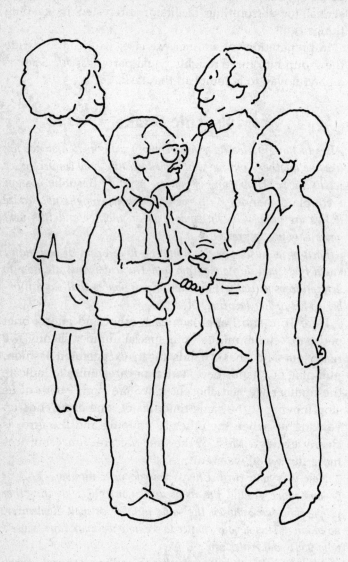

Psychic Shake

on the special number and that the three groups are clearly separated from each other around the room. This silly game serves to divide the group up somewhat randomly for the next activity, which we call

Commons

Great! Now that you know how psychic you can be, we are going to try an exercise in group sensitivity. First of all, each of the three groups is going to spend a few minutes deciding on a sound and a movement that demonstrates the combined energy in their group. Whatever it is, you just need to make sure everyone knows how to do it. We'll get back to you when you are ready. . . .

We then go around the room when the groups look ready and have each group demonstrate their particular creation. After we have seen what they have to offer, we have the other two groups practice what the presenting group has done just to let them see the total effect. This then lays the groundwork for the final test.

All right, you have seen each of the groups demonstrate its own combination of sound and movement to characterize the energy in that group. Now we will see how tuned in we all are to the energy in the group as a whole.

Each group needs to huddle up and independently decide which of the three demonstrations we have just seen best represents the energy in our whole group right now. No cheating! When each group has intuitively decided on its best guess, we will return to the center of the room and on the count of three see if we all agree.

When we get things back together and all three groups are sounding off at once, it is quite an effect. On occasion all three groups *do* pick out the same combination of sound and movement and the whole room erupts in delighted surprise. It is even more fun, however, when we don't agree, and end up taking two or three stabs at

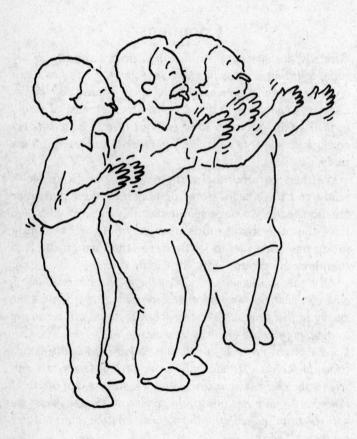

Commons

"tuning in." Most often we agree to disagree after a while, each group secretly still believing it had the best one to start with! We never were very psychic anyway. . . .

When time permits, we follow that game with one that has everyone searching for "the answer." We call it *Prui*. With the group gathered around close we talk for a minute about what we are all seeking—you know, the Prui!

Prui

Now that we have demonstrated our skills (or lack of them) in tuning in to each other, we want to give you the chance to find that which we all desire most—the Prui. As seekers blinded by ignorance and habit, we rarely find what is most important to us, and this game will give us a chance to practice doing just that. Here is how it works.

As one who is searching for the answer to life, I go around shaking hands with whomever I encounter and say, "Prui?" If the person I meet is also a seeker, he or she will respond, "Prui?" and I know I must keep on seeking. If, however, when I say "Prui?" the other person is silent, then I have found the one I seek—because, as we all know, those who don't know, speak, and those who know, don't speak. Know what I mean?

When I find the Prui, then I hold on with one hand and leave the other hand open for the next seeker to find as I become enlightened and join with the Prui. (That means I can open my eyes and remain silent from then on. We are all blinded with ignorance to start with, remember?)

So put your hands out in front of you to help you find your way around, start asking for the Prui, and keep your eyes closed at all times until you find the true Prui. We will be sure to keep you all in a safe area so that you don't prui the chairs, tables, or walls. And remember, no false Pruis out there! You are all seekers until you find the silent one and become one with the Prui yourself.

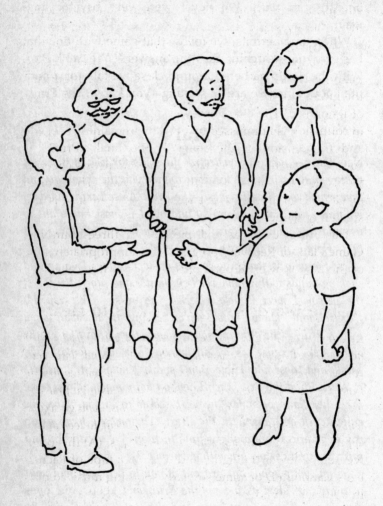

Prui

After everyone begins milling about like lost sheep, we pick one person to become the Prui and, whispering quietly in his or her ear, tell him or her to stand still, open his or her eyes and hands, and remain silent for the others to discover.

Gradually the seekers begin to latch on to the Prui, expanding the chain of "enlightened ones" and reducing the number of lost souls wandering about in the darkness of ignorance. The effect of fewer and fewer voices raised in confusion is not missed by even the remaining seekers, and the tension in the room as the final "Prui?" is sounded is generally released in a spontaneous cheer as all of the "lost ones" find their way home. The symbol of all becoming one is not lost either, even if it is not spoken of aloud. . . .

This brings us to the final piece of the three-hour New Game Plan for Recovery program. It is, appropriately, one of the most powerful parts of the process. It is called

The Words You Most Want to Hear

As our final activity of the evening, we need you to find a partner so that we can give you a parting gift. Stand with your partner in front of you and decide which of you will go first in this exercise and which will go second. Those who go first will move around the room in a moment while those who go second will remain where they are. Now take a moment to look at and appreciate your partner and then close your eyes. (At this point we quietly lower the lights and turn on a tape of Pachelbel's Canon in D or some similarly soothing music to play in the background.)

As you stand there with your eyes closed, we want you to think about the words you would most want to hear from someone close to you. Hear the words of appreciation, praise, or love that would mean the most to you right now and let that phrase

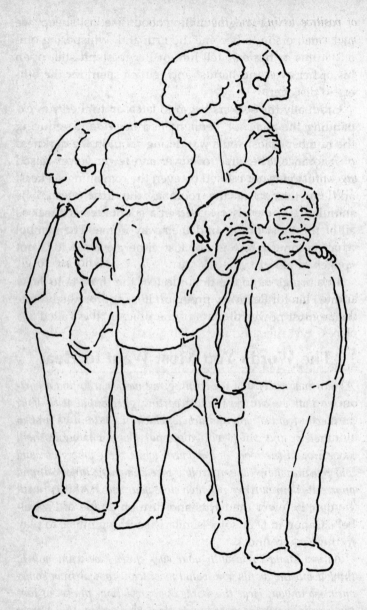

The Words You Most Want to Hear

of positive feeling and thought repeat itself over and over in your mind.

And now we want the one who is to go first to open your eyes, lean forward, and whisper the words you most want to hear into your partner's ear as if you were saying them to yourself. The one who is to go second should stay with eyes closed and listen. Then when you have finished, the one who is first should move around the room and quietly share the words he or she most wants to hear with the other people who are standing with their eyes closed.

When a few minutes have gone by and the ones going first have had a chance to share their message with most of the others standing still and listening, we ask them to return to their partners and stand once again with their eyes closed. Now it is the turn for those who are to go second to remember the words *they* most want to hear and to share them with their partner and the others as in the beginning. By the time we call them back to their places, each person has been bathed in a sea of support and love. The occasional quiet tears of joy are evidence of the lasting effects.

With partners back together again, we ask them to hear once again the words that surround them and know that they are true. We have them open their eyes and take a moment to give thanks to their partner for the gift they have received.

We leave a few moments for people to gather themselves back together as the lights come back up and then we move to the center of the room to say goodbye. . . .

As we get ready to go, we want to thank you for trusting us with your energy, playfulness, and joy. We couldn't do this without you. You have been a pleasure to play with and we encourage you to take this experience with you to share with others you know and love.

Before we go, however, we do have an important question to ask you. Having spent these past few hours with you we think you know the answer,

"WHAT DO YOU LIKE ABOUT YOURSELF?"

". . . EVERYTHING!!!"

Great! We do, too!

Thank you and good night.

10

Facilitating Fun

*Silly, originally, did not mean inane and stupid. It meant
four things: blessed, prosperous, happy, and healthy.*
DR. STEVE ALLEN, JR.

H aving introduced you to the activities which make
up The New Game Plan for Recovery, our goal is
that you share them with others. "Hug Tag" just doesn't
generate the same energy when you are playing by yourself. We have found over the years, however, that *what*
we do doesn't matter as much as *how* we do it—especially
when the people we are playing with have some doubts
about themselves, us, and (to begin with) the whole experience of play. Therefore, we would like to share with
you in this chapter some of the lessons we have learned
about facilitating play with groups of people of all sizes,
ages, attitudes, and agendas.

Planning

One of the most important aspects of facilitating play with groups of people emerges before you ever ask for their attention. Proper planning, having a sense of what you want to accomplish and how, can free your attention and energy for the action at hand. It may seem contradictory—how does one plan for spontaneity?—but the fact remains that it works.

On more than one occasion when caught on the spur of the moment (and realizing now why they call it a "spur") by a request for "some fun things," we have found our thoughts moving more toward the strange sensation in the pit of the stomach than toward the perfect play activity. Planning may include more than just what *you* do, too, as an example from our painful past will illustrate.

We are primarily speaking here of times when you are called on to *lead* others in some specific context. The situations in which you are part of a play community, large or small, and out to have fun yourself do not require the same sort of prior planning and attention to detail. But even in such cases, everyone stands to benefit as you increase your skill in having a good time.

Planning begins by knowing what you are getting yourself into. Our biggest lesson on that theme came when we were asked by a friend to facilitate some "enjoyable interaction" in his "History of Rock and Roll" class at a large university. We had by that time done numerous "gigs" in a variety of settings and were happy to oblige him.

On the appointed day we searched out his classroom—make that his auditorium—and walked into a room filled with some 500 college students more interested in the Beatles than Beethoven (but both were considered history by that time). The seats were elevated above a stage and we had to hook up to microphones to be heard. When time came for the class to start, our "friend" slapped us on the back, moved up to the fourteenth row and waved us into action.

The first problem was that he had apparently not prepared his class for this change of focus. As we started, several students visibly checked their watches and asked their neighbors if this was in fact the right class.

After we got underway with our carefully planned presentation, the realization spread that this was definitely *not* about rock 'n' roll and was probably *not* going to be on the test! By our fourth flat joke the exodus began as a goodly proportion of the students flipped their books shut, grabbed their backpacks, and headed for the door. The others stayed, we now assume, out of pure curiosity rather than compassion for the two presenters sweating it out on the stage. Comedians have a saying for rough shows, "I died in Cleveland." We were well into our death throes by ten minutes into our routine.

We made it through somehow. Probably half of the students hung around and participated by the time it was over. Our friend was delighted with the results and the ones who stayed probably got some mileage from the experience when they reached the student lounge later on for lunch. We were devastated.

Never again! College students are impossible! Maybe we shouldn't be doing this stuff after all. Oh, the shame of it! (Maybe they didn't catch our names!) Thank goodness we had each other to blame.

We wish no such experience on anyone. We did, however, live to play another day—even with college students at that same large university. And *their* reviews put us at the top of the list. The difference was that they were studying what we were presenting, they knew what was coming, and what we did *might* have been on the test. (That it wasn't did *not* influence their ratings of us!)

Suffice it to say: Know your audience and be sure *they know you*! A corollary to that principle is to always leave a suitable way out for those who simply aren't up to what you are doing. Hook whom you can and let the others slip quietly away.

The more participation you have from those who are there, the better energy you build for having a good time. (Our technique for spectators will be covered in the section on Encouraging.) Accept that most people will experience resistance to you at first. Then forget it in order to concentrate on the response you *are* getting from the group.

This is where planning a presentation comes in. We are much more at ease ourselves when we have a clear agenda of the activities, games, and exercises we want to share and a rough approximation of the time it will take to do so. Our general principle is to plan what we think will fit in the time allotted, then have two or three alternate activities in mind for special circumstances.

We also check with each other as we go along to insure we are matching up well with the needs and energy of the group. Finally, we also spend some time afterward in assessing how we did—what worked, what didn't, and what we might do next time.

As you get more experience leading, you will develop a more accurate sense of what will fit—in tone and time—for the context you anticipate. Our "plan" may be only on the back of a business card, but it can be a lifesaver when we need it. The pattern of activities in the previous two chapters is our generic favorite—feel free to improvise.

Modeling

Since play is, for adults, a somewhat uncomfortable activity when they aren't in control of it, you must actively model what you want to evoke in your participants. Being willing to have fun, be foolish, make mistakes, laugh, and play lets the folks you are leading know that they won't be alone if they take the risk of joining in.

One reason we like to work as a team is that, between the two of us, we can directly demonstrate the process, activity, or result we want them to engage in. Besides, two of us can keep the group's attention focused more easily as we present the next task.

The more concrete, clear, and visible you can be with what you are doing, the more likely it is that your audience will go along with what you are trying. The more congruent you are in expressing your own enjoyment of what you do, the more likely your audience will be attracted to what you are offering. We thoroughly enjoy what we do and that feeling is infectious. We also have a combined mental age of seven and a half, and it shows.

Be enthusiastic, but leave room for those who, at first, aren't. *Have fun*, it proves to some that fun is possible. *Demonstrate what you want people to do*; an action truly is worth a thousand explanations. *Allow for mistakes*—yours and others'—it makes things safe for those who are concerned about such things. *Practice what you preach*, an experienced player is a more attractive model for others to emulate. *Join in when you can* even as you monitor, encourage, pace, insure safety, and plan for the activity to follow.

Encouraging

We are two wild and crazy guys at times, and even *we* need some encouragement and permission when someone else is leading us in play. It is quite a risk for many people to let their hair down and their "childishness" show in full view of twenty (or two hundred) others. Our style is to be very supportive and encouraging when inviting people to play with us.

We do our best to find a way for anyone and everyone to participate in some capacity that fits their comfort zone. The New Games folks talk about changing the game to fit the players rather than the other way around. We heartily agree, and make every effort to convey that message to those with whom we play.

In an infinite number of ways, we can change what we do on any one occasion. We might change the rules, the roles, the goals, the boundaries, the scoring, the metaphor, the movement, the materials, the teams . . . you get the idea? We may even make a game out of finding new excuses not to play. Whatever works!

Our toughest line is for those who want to watch without joining in. We warn them that players are admitted free, but spectators pay $25! That rarely gets someone up who just isn't ready yet, but it does get them to think twice about it.

Ultimately we trust that those who stay just to watch must be getting something out of it or they would move along on their own. If they hang around, however, they can expect *at least a couple* of personal invitations to join in.

With certain activities there are those who will hold back. Our encouragement might take the form of slightly adjusting what they have to do in order to put it within their reach. Sometimes it means shifting the role from being the one in the center to being someone in support.

It is important to find a way for each person to feel a part of the action, even if he or she prefers a rather small part to begin with.

We are particularly careful to include anyone who by reason of age, disability, or other difference may be likely to feel a greater degree of isolation, discomfort, or hesitation. We may not have them do exactly what others are doing, but there is always a way to bring them into the action.

Along these same lines, certain activities are not appropriate for those with injured backs, ankles, etc. We do take care to identify such situations and make adjustments when necessary. On occasion those who are just plain hesitant have become our assistants and co-leaders. *That* generally encourages them to blend in better the next time!

We do give permission *not* to participate, though, even as we invite people to take a risk and jump in. In any case, where we see someone in distress, obviously uncomfortable, or truly reluctant to respond, we intervene in order to validate their feelings and make sure they are *not* pressured into something they are not ready to take on. That sort of pressure is often what they experienced all too many times growing up, and it is behind their hesitation in the present. The freedom to participate *or not* is part of the "voluntary" element in play, which is so essential to a rewarding experience.

In addition to participation, we also encourage the liberal use of imagination, humor, and creativity in order to have fun. The best way to do that is, of course, through modeling (did we talk about that?).

When we present activities or games we make an effort to "juice" them up as much as possible. Compare the effect of "Say something good about yourself to your partner" to the impact of all of the hoopla we generate (thanks to watching Matt Weinstein do his stuff!) with

What Do You Like About Yourself?—apples and oranges, brain freeze, Dragons of Doubt, sixty-second time limits—come on, already!

The fun of it all *does* seem to have something to do with the craziness factor, however, since as kids we were sane enough to be a lot crazier than we allow ourselves to be as adults.

A more subtle form of encouragement (and probably the best kind) is that generated from within the participants themselves. When we do a good job of planning and pacing (we will talk about that next), the success of each activity contributes to their investment in the next one.

We have heard from many New Game Plan players (fortunately *after* the whole thing was over) that at the beginning they were about as enthusiastic as a sloth on a slow day. Some even admit to having felt downright hostile as we'd got underway. "I dare you to make *me* feel good with all of this kid's stuff. I'm already in a positive frame of mind—I'm *positive* this ain't going to work!"

The ones we hear that from, however, are those who tell us with a note of awe in their voices and a glow of joy in their faces as they give us a handshake or a hug at the end of the session. They can't quite figure out how it happened, but they are ecstatic former skeptics and they want us to know it. That is *always* encouraging to us!

Essentially, we encourage people to take a risk and be willing to play the fool if need be in search of the playful energy of the Inner Child. We even specifically give permission to make mistakes, then make a few ourselves (sometimes even on purpose) in order to confirm our offer. The participants seem to have fun pointing them out to us.

Pacing

We are always aware of the energy level in the groups we work with (painfully so on occasion). The secret to a satisfying experience for the participants is to insure that we begin where *they* feel comfortable, shift their energy gradually into a higher level, then move from the peak of any one activity to the foothills of the next one until it is time to come down on the other side of the "range" for a rest. Avoiding boredom on one side and anxiety on the other is essential if the "flow" experience is to last.

A good job of pacing requires us to be sensitive about when to move on and what to move to. It means not getting ahead of ourselves or hanging on to the action too long. It involves a certain rhythm of action, interaction, and reflection that carries the group from one activity to the next in such a way as to have them feel "Yeah, that was fun, what's next?"

It can become a game in itself for us, a level of involvement that approximates a dance with each other and the entire group simultaneously. Perhaps that is part of the reason that, after hundreds of times of introducing and playing the same basic games, each time there is again a quality of "the first time." It is hard to convey in specifics, but when things are clicking it is impossible to ignore.

One very fundamental guideline is to *begin quickly slowly. Say what???* What we mean is that we work from the very first moment to engage our group directly. Our introduction, our jokes, our conveying a sense of empathy and acceptance, anticipation and excitement, all are designed to connect right away with those we are addressing. In our actions, however, we are careful to start slowly with activities and games that people will feel comfortable with and that engage them sometimes before they even know it.

Our typical "introductions" activity gets them up out of their chairs and talking to and touching a number of "strangers" within minutes. *The action, however, is only the means to another end* as far as the participants go, that of helping *us* out so that we are not the only silly looking people running around the room. This basic guideline suggests that you take advantage of the group's goodwill and willingness to play its part initially in order to overcome any underlying resistance and reluctance.

The beauty of playful experiences is that soon the *intrinsic* pleasure that results is the reward that motivates further engagement and involvement. Once that motivation is kindled, our role is simply to channel it in ever more satisfying directions.

Another principle we use regularly is to *allow enough time—but not too much*! Got that? What we mean here is to monitor each activity so that even as you introduce it you are sensing precisely when the group is ready to begin. We allow enough time for people to understand the directions before we get into the action. Puzzled looks, whispers among the group members, questions about what we just said, people running from the room—all these indicate it is not yet time to say "Hit it!"

Once the activity is underway, we want there to be a sense that everyone is involved and that most—but not necessarily all—will have had a chance to contribute. In certain settings we want to catch the energy at the peak before it begins to slip away, so we present another "New Game!" In others, we want more space for exploration, problem solving, or reflection by the group itself. In any case, depending on our goals, we use appropriately chosen activities to regulate the pace, rather than sheer boredom or exhaustion.

Finally, *in order to monitor the group we have to monitor ourselves*. When we notice a twinge of "when will this be over?" or a trace of "how much longer?", we move on.

We often find ourselves sending silent signals across a crowded room when our gut reaction says it is time for a change. It helps to make for an enchanted evening.

Pacing is a sort of "controlled flexibility." It gets easier with practice, and being good, encouraging models ourselves with an effective plan makes that practice much easier and more rewarding.

Insuring Safety

A constant focus and responsibility for anyone leading activities of these sorts is to insure safety for all concerned. When people accept an invitation to play, they do so with the implicit trust that what occurs will be to their benefit, not harm. As we have seen, one of the reasons play is so difficult for many is the history of inappropriate behavior, pain, and abuse that accompanied them through childhood. We consider it our responsibility to prevent any recurrence of such situations when others play with us.

As we go through The New Game Plan for Recovery we must be alert to conditions that might cause injury or pain physically, mentally, emotionally, or socially. While no one can completely control what happens to anyone, even oneself, it is possible and appropriate to anticipate the possible outcomes of what we do and to minimize the dangers to the best of our ability.

The most obvious of the areas needing our attention is the possibility of physical injury as a result of our activities. One reason we have not had such a problem occur is that we take that responsibility seriously and set limits openly and clearly to maintain safety.

When an activity requires or suggests rapid movement around the room or yard or park, we alert people to the boundaries and the obstacles that exist. If the exercise involves participants' putting themselves at some risk of falling—as *Willows in the Wind* does—we are careful to give detailed instructions *and* to monitor directly how things are going all along. For the games requiring closed eyes, we are constantly moving around the area to keep anyone from wandering into dangerous territory.

We watch for unsafe footing (even high heels), "traffic" jams, and obstacles that might get in the way of an unsuspecting player. Anytime the energy level of the group or of some individuals goes beyond what we feel comfortable with, we intervene. We may divert, caution, contain, limit, or change the game, but we take action to insure safety—that way we don't have to use *our* insurance!

Mental and emotional safety is, of course, as important as physical safety, if not more so. Recovery from a bump or a scrape is a question of time. Recovery from a bruised ego or battered spirit is a much more complex process.

Since we are encouraging people to revisit their vulnerable childhood consciousness, we must assure them they will be well treated while they are there. At the first signs of teasing, ridicule, shaming, and the like we move in to restore balance and trust. While we have never had a real problem in this area, we stay alert to the possibility of a "first time."

Since our whole goal is to bring people together, we work especially hard to incorporate everyone into the action. While there may be obvious distinctions between people to begin with, by the time we have moved into the play world, those differences seem to disappear. There are no CEO's, lawyers, custodians, laborers, housewives, or professors among a bunch of ten-year-olds. Barriers of all sorts seem to melt in the process of playing together and we are attentive to what it takes to keep it that way.

The goal of New Games is "cooperative competition" that engages everyone in a challenging yet safe and rewarding way. Pain, anxiety, shame, and fear disrupt this sort of playful interaction and interfere with its achievement. It is our responsibility to reduce them to a minimum whenever possible.

Releasing

The final principle we use as we lead these activities is *letting go*. There is a natural temptation to hold on to control, to hog the limelight, to hang on to action we initiate. We find that things go best when we actively give it away, however, and allow the natural creativity, energy, and enthusiasm of the group to be the focus.

Whenever possible we incorporate what the group has to offer in the very process of our presentation. We value the sort of dialogue that develops between us and the group. We encourage spontaneity and interaction among those we play with. We allow for changes in direction, timing, and even leadership when it will foster a more playful environment.

While we never really abdicate our position as facilitators (even as we join in the action), we do invite others to join us as leaders from time to time. Entering the "flow" is impossible if a rigid distinction between "us" and "them" prevails. As an ancient Chinese document, the Tao-te-ching, counsels, when the sage leads well, "The people say, we did it!"

Part of that "giving it away" is based on our experience of receiving from others and valuing their gifts. We want to keep "passing it on"! As we let go of controlling and enter into the "dance," we find ourselves blessed with an abundance of shared joy, delight, and pleasure many times greater than we could create on our own. In truth, *we couldn't do this by ourselves*!

Planning spontaneity, practicing what we preach, inviting involvement, controlling flexibly, competing cooperatively, and giving in order to receive, all of these seemingly contradictory behaviors help us to facilitate the creative paradox of play at work. Find some friends and try them out!

Just so you don't get the idea we have told you *everything* you need to know, we will further confuse you in the next chapter by throwing in a dozen or so alternative activities you can use to spice up any occasion and insure that it is best fit for those you are facilitating in play. See you there.

11

Variations on a Theme

He who laughs last, laughs best.
ANONYMOUS

He whose laughs last, laughs best.
MS. ANONYMOUS

He who laughs, lasts.
NOBODY KNOWS

The following activities are ones we use regularly in our New Game Plan presentations as alternatives to those already illustrated. In part, our choice depends on where we are (the surroundings), who we are playing with (new or experienced New Game planners), and how long it has been since we have played them. Sometimes the decision is absurdly simple. ("Did you bring along the balloons?" "But Tobin, I thought *you* were going to get them.")

In any case, you will see as we go along that we are paralleling the general pattern of chapters six and seven so that you can find suitable games for whatever segment of the process you may be in. Since these can be inserted anywhere, however, we will describe them as distinct exercises rather than in relation to each other as we tended to do in the earlier chapters.

One of our favorite ways to get a session started when we have a large open space, which lets us be more active, is by playing

Who Wants to Play?

For this game you will need several large soft Nerf balls, preferably in a variety of colors. Keep all but one of them out of sight as you introduce the game.

Hi there, as one way to get started this afternoon we would like to find out who wants to play. Any volunteers? Great, come on up here with us for a moment and we will explain what we are going to do next.

You have probably all played dodge ball at one time or another. This game is similar except that Claudia here is on one team and the rest of us are on the other. You see, Claudia raised her hand to indicate she wants to play and when she hits you with this nice, soft foam ball, you then raise your hand and keep it up to show you are a member of her team, and begin to play too. As more and more people get hit by a ball and raise their hands, it can get so exciting that in no time at all, everyone wants to play!

There is one rule you have to remember—when you pick up the ball to throw at someone else, you have to stay in that spot until you throw it. No running after someone to zap them, you must only throw the ball at them. Claudia's team (whenever she gets one) will need to work together to get everyone willing to play. The rest of us try as hard as we can to avoid getting touched by a ball. Watch out for tables, chairs, and plate glass windows as well as flying balls. Go get 'em, Claudia!

We let the game develop for a minute or so and then

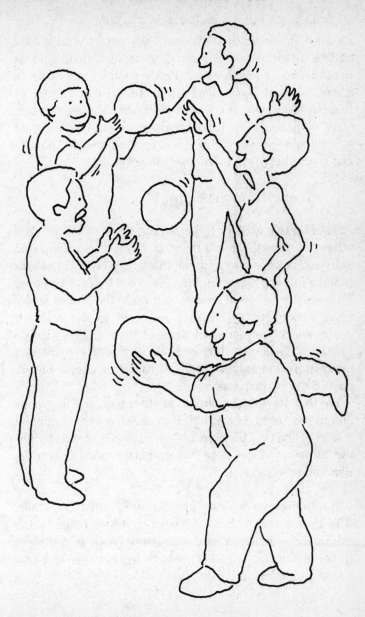

Who Wants to Play?

when everyone's attention is on the person with the ball, we start throwing in additional balls until we have four or five or more sailing around the room creating more people who "want to play." Pretty soon we are down to a few die-hard dodgers who bite the dust in a flurry of foam projectiles. You would be amazed at how much screaming, scurrying, and skulduggery can be generated by one silly game. When it's over, in any case, no one can claim they didn't "choose" to play. . . .

2×4's

An alternative activity to get strangers to talk with each other (we sometimes call them 2×4's) is to get them into pairs and ask them to find one thing they both did as kids to have fun and one thing they each did that was unique. This activity is a good lead-in later on to the *Guided Replay* visualization, since it means they get to think about, share, and be reminded of some of the activities kids do as part of their play life. It is also a positively oriented interaction that leaves plenty of room for choice on the part of the participants.

We then have each pair join another pair, and in groups of four have each partner introduce *the other one's* childhood games of choice. This expands the circle of "friends" without focusing on the more conventional aspects of occupation and roles, etc.

Another exercise for groups of four is called *Trust Falls*. It is a good way to build up trust in others while taking on an individual risk and succeeding with it. Safety is important in this one, so thorough instructions and adequate monitoring are essential.

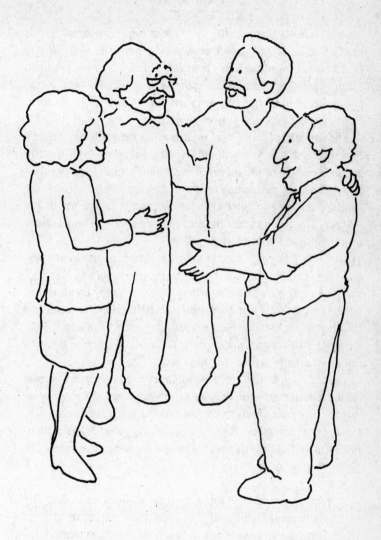

2×4's

Trust Falls

We are going to learn a little more about being supported in this next exercise, so will someone in each group who is willing to take a small risk please raise your hand. Fine. Now we need two "supporters" of approximately the same height to stand a couple of feet behind the volunteer and one "coach" to stand in front of and facing the person going first.

The supporters stand next to each other facing the volunteer's back, put one foot forward and one foot back, and bend slightly at the knees. They should bring their hands up in front of them, palms forward, with arms bent and prepare to gently catch the "faller" on the back just as he or she begins to lose his or her balance. The coach stands in front to make sure everyone is lined up straight and ready for the fall.

The ones "falling" should hold their arms across their chest and keep their body straight at all times as they slowly lean back into the supporters' hands. When they are ready, they call out "Ready to fall!" Then they wait until the supporters call out "Fall!" before making their move. After each little "fall," the supporters can move back a short distance to allow the one falling to go a little further the next time.

You will know you have gone far enough when the person falling squeaks involuntarily as he or she passes the point of no return. The coach makes sure everyone is ready before each fall. Go as far as the volunteer feels comfortable going before switching roles and giving the next person a chance to experience the "thrill" of support.

A variation activity for a group of eight is called the *Strength Bombardment* and it is especially useful in groups where the participants know each other from earlier interactions.

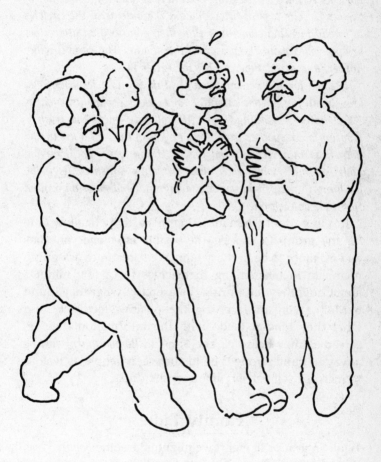

Trust Falls

Strength Bombardment

For this activity we need one volunteer to stand in the center of the circle. The task of the people on the outside of the circle is to briefly mention something that they admire, find attractive, or appreciate about the person in the middle. The more specific, honest, and direct they can be, the better it is.

The job for the person receiving this positive feedback is to keep breathing, listen carefully, and avoid comments such as "You gotta be kidding," or "If you only knew the truth." Appropriate responses from those of you in the center are to nod your head in agreement and to say "thank you" or "I'm glad you like that" when each other person is finished. Begin by listening to the person you are facing now and move on around the circle as each one finishes.

It is important when initiating this activity to allow time for the group to process the results after everyone has had a chance to be in the center. We sometimes ask group members to talk among themselves for a few minutes about how they felt during the exercise: what they found harder, giving or receiving the positive feedback, and what they tended to do with the information they received as they heard it. The *Strength Bombardment* can be a way to build stronger bonds between people as well as to increase self-esteem among individuals.

Family Time

While in groups of eight, we might take some *Family Time*. We ask the group members to huddle together and come up with a gesture and a name for their particular group. Whatever they think best represents the energy of their group or "family" at this time is fine (as long as they aren't all "rebels," in which case the gesture may need to be censored).

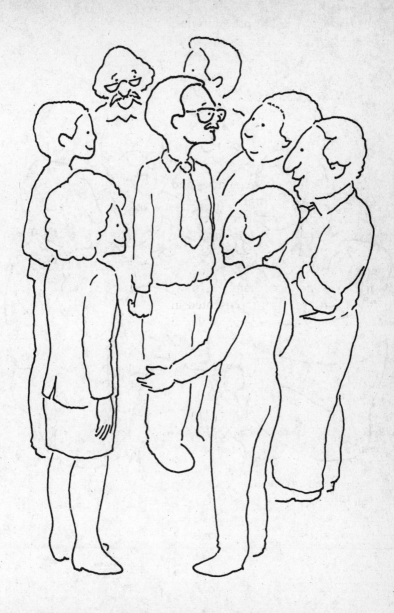

Strength Bombardment

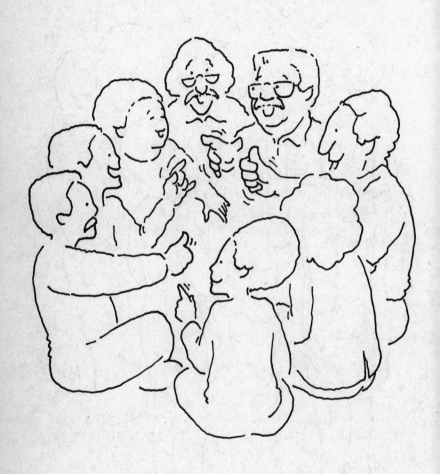

Family Time

When they are ready, we go around the room to let them share what they have come up with for everyone's benefit. We let them know that their "high-sign" is a way of signifying membership in their group and can be used at dinnertime, in elevators, staff sessions, and elsewhere to establish contact with a "brother or sister" and totally confuse anyone who is an "outsider."

Group Juggling

For groups from ten to sixteen or so in size, this is another "introductory" game we use from time to time. You will need those same large foam balls we used earlier, some tennis balls, beanbags, or the like to toss around the circle. Here's how it goes:

All right, everyone circle up and we will teach you a fascinating way to learn everyone's name in no time at all. I have a ball here and I am going to toss it to Joe and say his name out loud as I do. He will then toss it to someone else in the circle that he knows and call out his or her name as he does it. If he doesn't know anyone, then he can ask someone what his or her name is before throwing him or her the ball.

Remember who threw it to you and who you toss it to when it is your turn. Don't toss it to someone who has already had a turn, and the last person should throw it back to me. Here we go—Joe!

When the ball comes back to me after making it around the circle, I run through the sequence again for practice and then once in reverse. As an unexpected challenge, I then send it through one more time followed by about three other balls that I have hidden nearby just for such an occasion. When they are all sailing through the air (and rolling on the ground) at once, it can be a pretty overwhelming sight! At the end when I check for names, invariably no one has learned much more than before, but they have had a good time nonetheless.

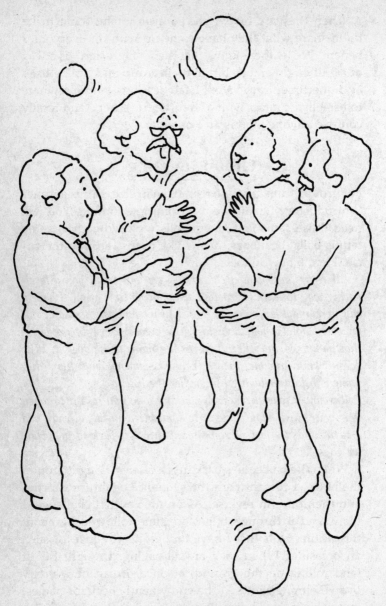

Group Juggling

Moving right along, we have a game that follows well on the heels of *Car Car*, from chapter 9. We call it

Convoy

After people have the idea about the basic *Car Car* game, we combine it with a chase sequence to get the advanced version. *For all you Burt Reynolds fans, we want to introduce you to* Convoy. *Beginning with everyone in their "vehicle," we will designate a "chase car" whose job it is to gently make contact with any other vehicle it can catch while moving around the room. It then joins up with that car by hooking on to the shoulders of the captured driver to make a "convoy" and the two joined cars* (with drivers) *go off in search of the next victim—I mean vehicle—until everyone is hooked onto the convoy.*

The captured car always becomes the lead car of the convoy which hooks on behind. Remember, cars are blind on their own, only drivers can see, but once they hook on to the convoy they can open their eyes—all except *for the* lead *car—so that they can enjoy the chase. Let's see how long it takes to get this convoy home. . . .*

An alternative and entertaining way to divide a large group up into two or three roughly equal groups is to play

Nighttime Barnyard

The number of groups is a direct result of the number of animals introduced in the beginning.

It's time to get organized around here, and the best way we know to do that is to see what kind of a group we have here. You are all acquainted with some typical barnyard inhabitants such as chickens and pigs. What kind of sounds do chickens make? How about pigs? Fine! Now, we know that one of these two animals happens to be your favorite. We also know that birds of a feather flock together and pigs prefer pigs

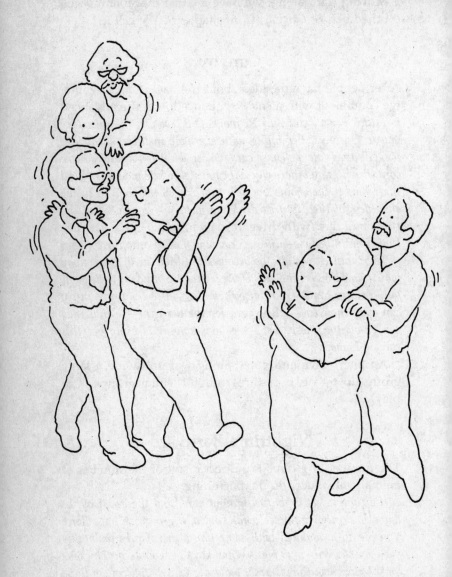

Convoy

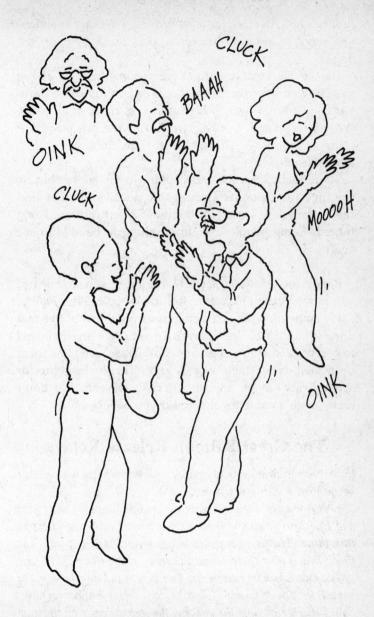

Nighttime Barnyard

in their digs. All you have to do now is by clucking or oinking find everyone else who belongs to your breed. Not too bad, huh?

Oh, by the way, be sure to keep your guards up as you move around the room, since this is called Nighttime Barnyard *and you do have to have your eyes closed at all times. We will keep watch to make sure that no one gets plucked or steps in anything. Go get 'em! Here chick, chick . . . soooooooweee!*

There really isn't too much point to this game, but by the time the chickens and pigs or ducks and cows find their comrades, some real bonds of friendship are being forged. Some people will do anything to be able to see again.

Ready for a *balloon blowout*? We often run a series of games we learned from Karl Rohnke's book, *Silver Bullets*, using some medium-sized balloons from the local five and dime (that's $5.10 these days). To start, we give balloons to everyone, one to a customer, and have them blow them up *without* tying them off in a knot. This is the setup for a relay race unlike any you have ever seen. We don't really have a name for it. Would you believe

The Great Balloon Release Relays

(Say that ten times quickly and you'll know why we haven't settled on a name for it yet.)

Everybody got their balloons blown up? Come on over here and line up in two (or three or four) nice, neat rows next to each other. The first person in line is at the starting point. The finish line is over there across the room where those chairs are.

The race is run by having the first person in line release his or her balloon, watch it until it lands somewhere on the floor (or table, light fixture, etc.), and then having the second person on the team run over to that spot, wherever it is, release his or her balloon,

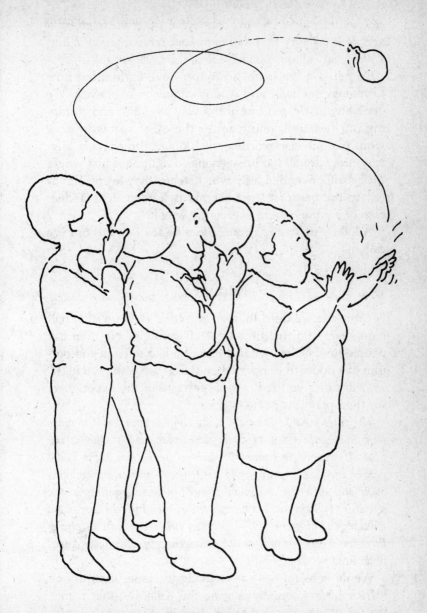

The Great Balloon Release Relays

etc., until we either run out of people or one of the teams man-
ages to get one of its balloons to land across the finish line.
Watch your balloons carefully! Ready, set, let 'em go!

To tell you the truth, we never have figured out how
to referee this wild and woolly explosion of activity. We
generally just stand out of the way shouting and stomping our feet until one team or the other seems to have
won. No one else worries much about the winners anyway; they are all too busy trying to figure out just where
their balloon ended up, which team they were on, or
where the bag of extra balloons is hidden. It is a clear
case of a game where everybody wins!

A follow-up to *The Great Balloon Release Relays* is one we
call

Popcorn

For this one we need to have everyone blow up their balloon again and this time tie it off securely. We then ask
people to visualize what it must be like to be at the bottom of a popcorn popper when things are going full blast.
In order to give them a real-life taste of the experience,
we then play this game.

The rules for this game are fairly simple. Your job is to make
sure that neither your balloon nor anyone else's touches the
floor after we begin bouncing them up in the air. Tobin and I
will be the floor monitors and alert you to any errant balloons
by quietly shrieking at the top of our lungs and pointing at the
offending balloon until someone gets it back into the air where
it belongs. The game will stop when either you hear us shriek
three times each, or we lose our voices entirely, whichever comes
first. Ready to pop? POP!

We demonstrate as we go along to insure that no one
thinks we are actually *popping* the balloons—that comes
later—but we often fail to tell them that we plan on adding another five or ten balloons to the mix just to keep

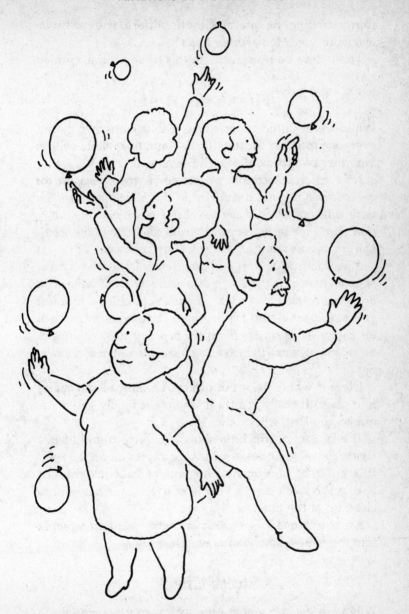

Popcorn

things exciting. Be careful with the shrieks, you really can lose your voice remarkably quickly. . . .

The "pièce de résistance" of this trilogy is one entitled

Fire in the Hole

When we get tired of chasing loose balloons, we gather everyone together for the "finale" and have them choose a partner of approximately the same height.

Now that you have your partner and your balloons, we are going to play a game called Fire in the Hole. *In demolition work with explosives, when the charge is set and ready to be blown up, the responsible party shouts out "Fire in the hole!" to warn anyone nearby of the impending explosion.*

All you have to do is set the charge between you—that's right, put one balloon right between your bodies at about bellybutton height—give out a loud cry of "fire in the hole!" and then just give each other a great big hug until the concussion tells you the charge has gone off! It's really very safe when you follow the instructions exactly. Do I have a volunteer for a demonstration?

(Here is where the art of picking a *willing* victim comes into play.) It really *is* a thrill when you finally get someone to go along with you.

The last act of this little show is a quick round of *Pick Up the Pieces*, the rules of which we improvise on the spot. It is amazing how many remnants of balloons you can find in the room even a year later if you aren't careful to clean up at the time.

An alternative large group activity we often squeeze into the New Game Plan is what we call a

Stress Check

When we get the whole group in one circle, we talk to them for a moment about stress in our culture, behavior,

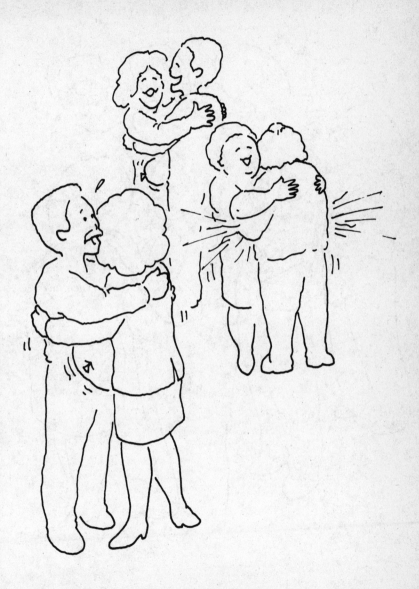

Fire in the Hole

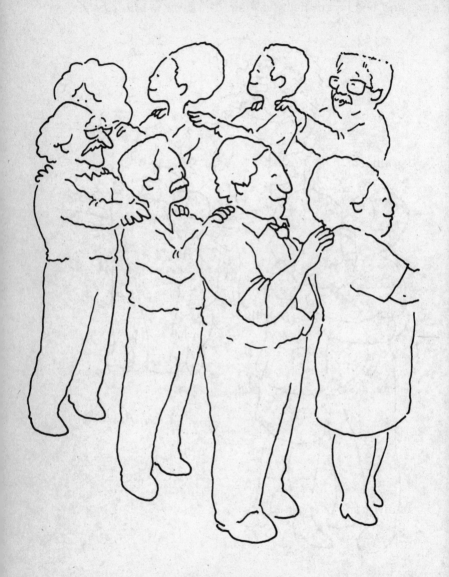

Stress Check

and body. We then get them to "check it out," making
sure we are in the circle *ourselves* when they do.

*We are going to give you a technique we know to help you
assess the level of stress in people you know and reduce that
stress all at the same time. To begin with we want all of you to
turn to the right. Fine. Now you probably know that the greatest level of stress is usually concentrated in the shoulders and
neck. Reach out to the person in front of you and gently check
out the tension level he or she is experiencing right now. Rub
gently but firmly to help loosen any tight muscles you may
discover. How does that feel?*

If people are lined up in a circle to begin with, of course,
when they turn to the right they have someone right behind them as well as in front. The chorus of ah's and oh's
is general confirmation that what they are giving is being
received as well. After a couple of minutes we make that
process more overt.

*Now, since there is a law of the universe that what you give
out is what you get, will everyone please turn the other way
and return the gift to the giver.*

*We generally recommend this exercise as a good way to pass
the time you spend waiting in line at the supermarket, post
office, and the like. Just don't tell them we told you to do this!
Feeling any better? We thought so.*

A concluding activity we use from time to time is called

Wrap Up

It is suitable for groups up to perhaps 50 or 75 in number.
Any group larger than that tends to take too long to complete the process. Beginning with everyone in the proverbial large circle, we station ourselves next to each other
and ask everyone to grasp hands with their neighbor.

*We would like to lead you in a little song and dance as our
final activity of the program. The words of the song go like this
(if you haven't heard the tune, make one up):*

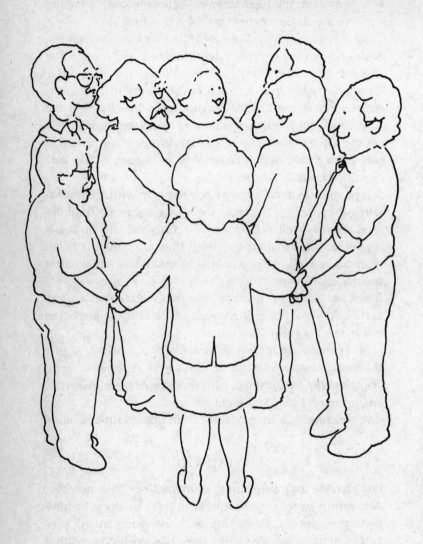

Wrap Up

Listen, listen, listen to my heart's song.
Listen, listen, listen to my heart's song.
I will never forget you, I will never forsake you.
I will never forget you, I will never forsake you.

One of us (never Tom) sings the song as the group begins to join in. We keep on repeating the song as the two of us let go of our hands and one of us moves toward the center of the room, leading the rest of the people on his side in that direction and then standing still. The other one of us begins to lead the rest of the group around the outside of the group in a spiral effect encircling those in the center.

Gradually the line of people begins to tighten up around the center point and we create a giant group hug, with everyone stretched at arm's length around those in the middle. As we get to the end and the circle is entirely rolled up, the one of us on the outside finishes up the song and lets everyone know that just about "wraps it up."

After we let the group experience what it is like to hug 40 (or 50, etc.) people at once, we tell them to hold on while we get them out of this mess. The one of us in the very center of the spiral then drops down under the outstretched arms of the tightly bound group and—pulling his neighbor out behind him—wiggles through the bodies until he reaches freedom. We generally start singing some other song (such as "Amen") as the great escape is accomplished and the group gradually unwinds itself from the center out ending up in the original large circle once more.

It is a good idea to practice this procedure with some willing friends before you try it out on a bunch of strangers. The singing is a big part of the effect, and not knowing which way to go can turn the exercise into a modern-day version of the Gordian Knot! When you get it right, however, the effect is marvelous.

One other activity we sometimes finish up with is called the

Vortex

This one is similar in some ways to the *Wrap Up*, but has its own special character and complications.

Beginning in a large circle with everyone holding hands, we introduce the exercise with a song (where have we heard *that* before?). The same song from the previous exercise works unless we have used it already, in which case we have another one handy. In any case, as we begin the song we start the group moving slowly to the left. One of us then lets go of the person on his left, and moves just inside the circle leading the others behind him at a slightly increased rate. We create a kind of clockwise spiral again, but this one is led from in front toward the center instead of from outside around everyone else.

After several circles, the leader gets closer and closer to the center of the spiral and it appears that there is no way out. But at the last moment, just as he is about to run out of room, the leader turns sharply to the left and begins to thread his way out of the spiral by moving between the rings that have been created. The result is that everyone passes everyone else as they spiral into the center and back out of it.

Once back out of the "vortex," the leader makes another turn, this time to the right, in order to bring the line back in the direction in which it began. Ultimately, unless things get "out of hand," the whole group passes by itself several times on the way back to the beginning point as the leader hooks back on to the person he let go of a few minutes before. The chance to say "hello and good-

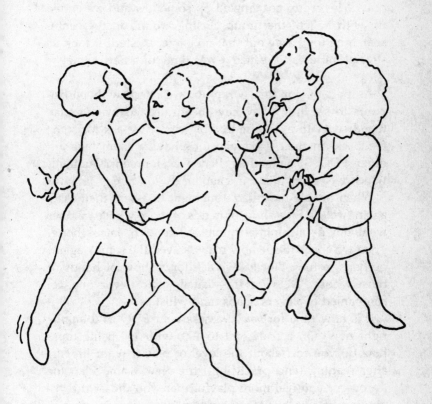

Vortex

bye'' to all of our newfound playmates is a unique way
to end the program, and the overall impact is delightful.

Just be sure you don't get carried away with yourself
and attempt this with two hundred people, as we did
once. The group got tangled up somehow and we ended
up with half of the group circling around in the center
searching for a way out that no longer existed. It took us
several minutes to realize it was time for a new game!

As part of our final wrap-up, we check with participants to see how they have been affected by our play
together. With everyone in a big circle, we ask for some
feedback on their experiences by having them take another PDQ. (That's their Play Development Quotient,
which we talked about in chapter 2.)

When people have had a moment to assess their PDQ
again, we ask for a show of hands of those whose number
went down—a minimal number, like zero, let us hope.
Then we check to see how many stayed the same—again,
perhaps, a few. Finally, we ask for a show of hands of
those whose PDQ went up—usually almost everyone, accompanied by cheers, claps, and whistles.

It is now time for *you* to assess your PDQ as it stands
right now. On a scale of 1 to 100, with 100 being tops,
how do you feel about the level of play in your life? If,
after reading (and practicing!) the New Game Plan for
Recovery, you feel more playful than you did at the beginning of this book, even potentially, you are on the
right road. If not, you can stop right here and find something more enjoyable to do with your time (since that is
our goal in any case). Either way, you have learned something valuable that you can apply right now in your life.
Finally, we always ask the group once again that most
important of questions which we advised them about in
the beginning. We want them to remember clearly ''What
do you like about yourself?''

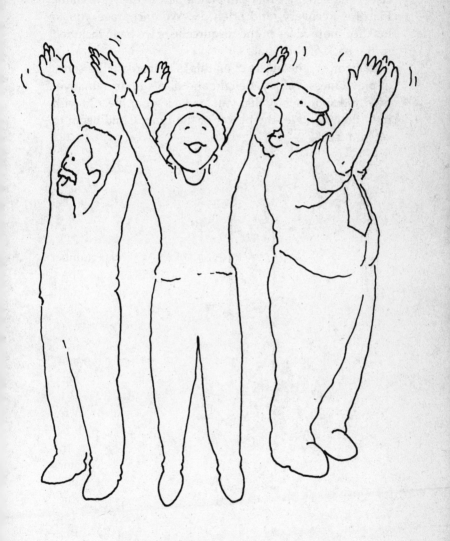

What Do You Like About Yourself?

There are, of course, innumerable other games, exercises, and activities that can play a part in the New Game Plan for Recovery, and often do. We encourage you to look for more ideas in the resource lists we have included in the back of this book.

Remember, the object of all this is to increase the sense of playfulness and joy, delight and pleasure, imaginativeness and spontaneity that you create in your life. Go with the "flow" and let the power of the Inner Child begin to set you free!

A Collection of
Quotations (Part 2)

If I had to live my life over again,
I'd dare to make more mistakes next time.
I'd relax.
I would limber up.
I would be sillier than I have been this trip.
I would take fewer things seriously.
I would take more chances.
I would take more trips.
I would climb more mountains, swim more rivers.
I would eat more ice cream and less beans.
I would perhaps have more actual troubles, but I'd have
* fewer imaginary ones.*
You see, I'm one of those people who live seriously and
* sanely hour after hour, day after day.*
Oh, I've had my moments.
And if I had it to do over again, I'd have more of them.
In fact, I'd try to have nothing else, just moments, one
* after another, instead of living so many years ahead of*
* each day.*
I've been one of those persons who never goes anywhere
* without a thermometer, a hot water bottle, a raincoat,*
* and a parachute.*
If I had it to do again, I would travel lighter than I have.
If I had to live my life over, I would start barefoot earlier
* in the spring and stay that way later in the fall.*
I would go to more dances.
I would ride more merry-go-rounds.
I would pick more daisies.
NADINE STAIR (AGE 80)

A sense of humor is the only divine quality of man.
SCHOPENHAUER

Play fuels your creativity,
Tickles your inner child,
And nurtures your soul.
CLAUDIA BLACK

The author of genius does keep to his last breath the spon-
taneity, the ready sensitiveness, of a child. . . .
DOROTHEA BRANDE

There is no cure for birth and death save to enjoy the
interval.
GEORGE SANTAYANA

Life does not cease to be funny when people die any more
than it ceases to be serious when people laugh.
GEORGE BERNARD SHAW

There is, in fact, no real ''spirituality'' (a much misun-
derstood term in these days) without the laughter which
a sense of humor brings.
HELEN LUKE

A smile is a curve that sets everything straight.
PHYLLIS DILLER

The dynamic principle of fantasy is play, which belongs
also to the child, and as such it appears to be inconsistent
with the principle of serious work. But without this play-
ing with fantasy no creative work has ever yet come to
birth. The debt we owe to the play of imagination is in-
calculable.
DR. CARL G. JUNG

Play is meeting challenges with skills for the sake of making that match.

DR. MCCALL

If you want to become more creative, remain in part a child, with the creativity and invention that characterizes children before they have been deformed by adult society.

JEAN PIAGET

A child, as well as an adult, needs plenty of Spielraum *. . . "free scope, plenty of room"—to move not only one's elbows but also one's mind, to experiment with things and ideas at one's leisure, or, to put it colloquially, to toy with ideas.*

BRUNO BETTELHEIM

You can discover more about a person in an hour of play than in a year of conversation.

PLATO

Explorations
in Play

12

Playing with Spirit

The sage is shy and humble—
to the world he seems confusing.
Men look to him and listen.
He behaves like a little child.
TAO-TE-CHING

We have described in numerous ways the unique energy and spirit we often see in children. We have suggested that we can generate some of that energy in our own life as adults. In this chapter we would like to play with one final possibility.

Does our developing a more playful perspective in life do *more* than reduce stress and increase the level of health and happiness we experience? Is it possible that this drive to play, so clearly seen in children, is evidence of a spirit far more extensive and expansive than we might at first allow? Could we be made "in the image of God" in more fundamental ways than we imagine?

The qualities of the child—focused attention, creativity, curiosity, wonder, awe, faith, willingness to risk, love, and the like—may hold clues for us to the source of a greater mystery, the spirit of Life itself.

We would like to spend our final few moments together with you exploring the possible relationship between playfulness—joy—and a spiritual life.

Spirit is defined in Webster's New Universal Dictionary as "(a) the life principle, especially in man, originally regarded as an animating vapor infused by the breath, or as bestowed by a deity; (b) the soul." It is derived from the Latin, *spiritus*, meaning breath, courage, vigor, the soul, life. *Enthusiasm*, another word often used to describe the energy of the young, is related to the Greek word *entheos*, meaning "filled with God."

Perhaps the connection between the spirit, animation, and creativity of a child and the Spirit that is within and beyond us all is no coincidence. Perhaps as children, newly arrived in this world, we are closer to the Source from which we all come.

William Wordsworth's poem "Ode: Intimations of Immortality" offers eloquent expression to this perspective:

> *Our birth is but a sleep and a forgetting:*
> *The Soul that rises with us, our life's Star,*
> *Hath had elsewhere its setting,*
> *And cometh from afar:*
> *Not in entire forgetfulness,*
> *And not in utter nakedness,*
> *But trailing clouds of glory do we come . . .*

Masters of the Dream World

We are all familiar with the world of dreams. Even if we don't recall the ones we have during the night, we are sometimes aware of the dreams that catch our attention during the day. At times, these visions can seem quite real. Fortunately or unfortunately—depending on the dream—we realize our misperception when we "wake up" and find ourselves in the "real world" again.

Children are masters of the dream world. They enter it at will and "make believe" with incredible power and perception. Even when they are not encouraged by caring adults, they generate fantasies rich in detail and extensive in scope. They incorporate, when available, the insights and inspirations of others, yet negotiate with fierce determination to insure that the outcome is what it's "s'posed to be." The worlds of their imagination have a clarity and coherence that are captivating even to those who are simply observers.

Their drive to engage in playful action and interaction is almost as strong as their need for food and shelter, and the nourishment they derive from such action is every bit as essential to their growth and development.

What if these essential skills of children, the honesty and innocence of perception, the power of imagination, the openness to innovation, the vitality and vibrancy of involvement, the ever present drive to the creation of meaning, are the qualities of Creation itself?

What if the amazing energy of the universe that sets stars in motion and galaxies to spin is reflected in the endless activity and intensity of the young?

What if even our notion of "reality" is just another level of dreaming, real enough during the experience of it, but one from which we may "awaken" eventually as we perceive still other realms and levels of existence?

For eons, the aboriginal people of Australia have survived in wilderness we can hardly conceive of by entering the "dream time" to track quarry along trails that are months old and to "smell" their way to pools of water hidden beneath the crusted earth. Perhaps the power and purpose of our "imagination" are greater than we might at first think.

The Game of Life

Evidence of this possibility comes to us from cultures and traditions ancient and modern, east and west, simple and sophisticated. Poets and prophets from time immemorial have called us to a vision of a larger life beyond this "world of dreams."

The contemporary game called Snakes and Ladders, for example, has its roots in the India of thousands of years ago when the dance of the universe was represented in the game of Leela. As described by an eminent scholar of the Sanskrit language, Harish Johari, in his introduction to a translation of the game,

> There is really only one Game, the Game in which each of us is acting out his role. The Game is Leela, the universal play of cosmic energy. . . . As with all games, here too there is a goal—an object to be attained. Because the essence of the player is his ability to identify, his only chance of "winning" the Game is to identify with that which is his Source. This is Cosmic Consciousness, the essence of pure Being which transcends time and space and knows no limits. The Game ends when the player becomes himself, the essence of play. This is Leela.

The goal of the game of life is achieved, then, when we once again recognize our essential unity with the universal energy that is the source of all things, however we choose to describe it.

Mystical traditions the world over have called on us to see through the "veils of illusion" that keep us from the experience of life "as it is" in its "fullness."

At one conference on the nature of the inner life, Lama Govinda, a Westerner who became a scholar and practitioner of Tibetan Buddhism, was outlining the stages on the path to enlightenment in that tradition.

In the question and answer period that followed his lecture, a participant stood and asked if there were any way to tell, any markers to indicate that one was actually making progress in the journey of the Spirit. Without hesitation and with a radiant joy manifest in his voice, Lama Govinda responded,

"Why certainly . . . happiness!"

The innocence and purity of the child has often been a metaphor for this experience, or "realization" in the deepest sense. As models of that sense of clear and enlightening energy and the delight in life that can accompany it, we know of no more accessible examples than that of children at play. And we *all* have been children who played. . . .

We see the connection between the child and the spiritual life also in this passage from Luke 18: 16–17, where we hear Christ saying,

> Let the children come to me, and do not hinder them;
> for to such belongs the kingdom of God. Truly, I say
> to you, whoever does not receive the Kingdom of God
> like a child shall not enter it.

And is it any surprise that those who have had an experience of profound transformation, in the Christian tradition as well as others, speak of it as being "reborn"?

A Child of the Universe

The musings of today's theoretical physicists sound strangely similar to these themes at times. Holography, entrainment, resonance, charm—the stuff of art, drama, and music—are now the province and language of scientists as well.

George Leonard, writing of the "new physics" in his book *The Silent Pulse*, describes the paradoxical state of harmony possible in those rare moments when we are in tune with the underlying rhythm of the universe:

> During those times, as we've seen in our stories, what we intend happens and what happens is what we intend. There is no waiting, since everything is already taking place. There is no unfulfilled desire, since desire itself dissolves on the ever-present instant of fulfillment. There are no chance events, since we are the architects of creation and all things are connected through us. Others around us (other universes) report that they, too, are affected. Miracles seem to happen, eventually seeming less like miracles than "just the way things are." The ego is not destroyed or distressed, as in schizophrenia, but transcended. Each of us, in this ultimate interplay, is like a god, omnipotent and omniscient. Does this mean we can fly or move mountains? It's impossible to say. But whatever happens is just what is intended. In the playground of reality, where the relationship between identity and holonomy is directly experienced, each of us is in the business of creating all of existence, effortlessly, on the wink of an instant.

What an eloquent description of the child at play! Do we dare consider it a possibility for us as full-grown adults? Imagine living life with little or no expectations, investing our energy fully in the activity at hand, becoming absorbed in the present moment and capable of feeling the total range of emotions we have available—all while retaining the sense of detachment and security that comes from knowing this is but another form of play. Imagine, with all the power and control we possess as "creators," acknowledging at the most basic level our own limitations and finiteness in relation to the greater power that truly sustains us.

Without surrendering our hard-earned knowledge in some hapless return to ignorance, without denying our extensive experience with the world as it is, without limiting ourselves to the trivial repetition of "childish" activities, we may yet be able to renew ourselves, to grow to greater levels of skill and grace in the ever expanding dance of life. This is what author Jean Houston refers to as "high play."

And when our own personal "dramas" get too intense, and we lose our balance and our path along the way, what more powerful call to a sense of freedom, joy, and serenity could there be than the realization that this world, too, may be but another dream in the infinite mind of God, one in which we are learning the lessons we need to learn in order ultimately to merge with the ongoing "flow" of creation.

We needn't idealize children and the life they lead in order to consider this thesis (though we *do* fall prey to that tendency at times). Nor need we try to actualize our absolute potential at all times. We need not even be "religious" in the conventional sense, to find grounds for this sort of "transformation."

Whether one's faith is in the "laws of nature," the God of a religious tradition, "a Higher Power," a Transpersonal Self, or the moving hand of Fate, the mystery that surrounds us remains the same. We are all children when it comes to comprehending Reality.

It is in the *experience* of life, the surrender to that which is greater than we are, the acceptance of that which is beyond our understanding, the willing engagement with that which presents itself to us in each moment, that we find our reward and fulfillment. This is the very essence of growing young again, of becoming a child of the universe.

What we are suggesting is simply that the Spirit that creates and sustains us, however we understand it, may be contained within each of us; may be as close as the dialogue we initiate with the powerful creative energy of our own Inner Child.

It is not, of course, the only source of wisdom, joy, and power. A balanced, healthy life requires us to honor *all* parts of ourselves, the child *and* the adult. It is when we willingly, actively, and openly acknowledge the energy of the Inner Child, however, that we make possible the development of a more meaningful "maturity," one at home in this world and any others that might be available.

As we attend to and affirm the childlike qualities that are our heritage and birthright, we are setting out on another stage of the journey to recovering a sense of the whole self, innocent *and* wise, expressive *and* experienced, full of wonder *and* awareness.

In freeing our Inner Child we free ourselves, coming in the end once more to our beginning and experiencing it again—with the energy and serenity of a child at play— for the first time.

By Virtue of Participation in a CELEBRATION of
The New Game Plan for Recovery
We, the Undersigned, Hereby Declare

to be a true and faithful, fully recognized

Free Child

In honor of such designation, said Celebrant is hereby authorized and encouraged to experience and express all the QUALITIES which are the birthright and heritage of the Free Child

Furthermore, said Designee is henceforth & forevermore empowered to laugh and cry, to create and grow, to make mistakes and let go, to dream (while sleeping and awake), to act (for real and just to kid around), and to feel, sense, savor, and celebrate the fullness of the world in which we live, ever remembering . . .

Curiosity Joy playfulness
FLEXIBILITY energy wonder
imagination TRUST
spontaneity humor
CREATIVITY
Honesty and Love

ITS NEVER TOO LATE
to have a happy childhood

Signed and sealed this ___ day of _____, ___.

© 1989
Tobin Quereau
Tom Zimmermann

Tobin Quereau   Tom Zimmermann

**Full-page, framable certificates are available from
Playmakers (see resource guide).**

A Collection of Quotations (Part 3)

When one has understanding, one should laugh, one should not weep.

HSUEH-T'OU

God works and man plays—or that is the way the scheme is set up and meant to be. I like it that way.

JOSEPH CHILTON PEARCE

I got into the ocean and played.
I played on the land too.
I also played in the sky.
I played with the devil's children in the clouds.
I played with the shooting star in space.
I played too long and years passed.
I played even when I became a tottering old man.
My beard was fifteen feet long.
Still I played.
Even when I was sleeping, my dream was playing.
Finally I played with the sun, seeing which one of us
    could be redder.
I had already played ten thousand years.
Even when I was dead I still played.
I looked at the children playing, from the sky.

TOZU NORIO (AGE 11)

I suspect this making of "nonsense" out of what is supposed to make sense is part of one of the great lessons of play—the child's growing aptitude to transform.

RICHARD LEWIS

There is more honest "belly laughter" in a Zen monastery than surely in any other religious institution on earth. To laugh is a sign of sanity; and the comic is deliberately used to break up concepts, to release tensions and to teach what cannot be taught in words. Nonsense is used to point to the beyond of rational sense.

CHRISTMAS HUMPHRIES

A laugh can be a very powerful thing. Why sometimes in life it's the only weapon we have.

ROGER RABBIT

It is the sense of humor that renders life a great deal more endurable than it would otherwise be, and much more amusing. Clearly humor is one of our greatest and earliest natural resources.

ASHLEY MONTAGU

Follow your bliss.

JOSEPH CAMPBELL

Maturity: among other things, the unclouded happiness of the child at play, who takes it for granted that he is at one with his playmates.

DAG HAMMARSKJÖLD

There are things that even the wise fail to do,
  While the fool hits the point.
Unexpectedly discovering the way to life in the midst of death,
He bursts out in hearty laughter.

SENGAI

*God alone is worthy of great seriousness, but man is made
God's plaything, and that is the best part of him.*

PLATO

*Children's playings are not sports and should be deemed
their most serious actions.*

MONTAIGNE

*Grow young with me!
The best is yet to be,
The last of life, for which,
   the first was made.*

AMENDED AFTER ROBERT BROWNING, RABBI BEN EZRA

*Daddy, I never, ever in my life, get enough time to finish
my play!*

JENNIFER QUEREAU (AGE 6)

RESOURCE A

People and Organizations

W e would like to introduce you to some people we have gotten to know personally over the years and some resources that we have found to be helpful in increasing our sense of playfulness, pleasure, and well-being.

We group them in our own fashion arbitrarily but nonetheless in hopes of making them accessible according to your needs. We cannot guarantee that by the time you read this they will all still be in business, in town, or in print; we hope you will find your way to the ones you want—or to others that we don't even know about yet.

In fact, we would like you to become a resource for us as well. Please feel free to let us know of your reactions to, experiences with, and comments on *The New Game Plan for Recovery*. Copies of your work on the exercises (save the originals!) or responses to the visualizations would be very helpful to us. Any favorite toys, games, or players you think we would like to know about also would be greatly appreciated. You can reach us at Playmakers as listed under *Organizations* below.

People

Stars from the Playing Field

Steve Allen, Jr., M.D.
8 La Grande Ct.
Ithaca, NY 14850
(607) 277-1795
physician, juggler

Peter Alsop, Ph.D.
P.O. Box 960
Topanga Canyon, CA 90290
(213) 455-2318
singer, songwriter, playful performer

Annette Goodheart, Ph.D.
P.O. Box 40297
Santa Barbara, CA 93140
(805) 966-0025
laughter therapist, workshop presenter

Joel Goodman, Ph.D.
The HUMOR Project
110 Spring St.
Saratoga Springs, NY 12866
(518) 587-8770
Director, The Humor Project

Ann McGee-Cooper, Ed.D.
Ann McGee-Cooper and Associate, Inc.
P.O. Box 64784
Dallas, TX 75206

(800) 477-8550
consultant on play, writer

Anne Robinson
2309 Shoal Creek Blvd.
Austin, TX 78705
(512) 472-4412
creativity consultant, trainer, writer

Karl Rohnke
Project Adventure
P.O. Box 100
Hamilton, MA 01936
(508) 468-1766
writer, workshop leader, kite flyer

Dr. O. Carl Simonton
Simonton Cancer Center
875 Villa de la Paz, Suite C
Pacific Palisades, CA 90272
(213) 459-4434
physician, writer, juggler

Matt Weinstein, Ph.D.
2207 Oregon St.
Berkeley, CA 94705
(415) 486-1244
President, Playfair Inc.
workshop presenter and consultant on play

Bruce Williamson
P.O. Box 11729
Albuquerque, NM 87192
(505) 293-3185
Director, Back to Nurture
workshop presenter and consultant on play

Playful Stars from the Recovery Field

Claudia Black, Ph.D.
Claudja, Inc.
1590 S. Coast Hwy.
Laguna Beach, CA 92651
(714) 497-3566
writer, therapist, trainer, workshop leader

Dr. Timmen Cermack
Genesis
1325 Columbus Ave.
San Francisco, CA 94133
(415) 346-4460
writer, therapist, workshop leader

Rokelle Lerner
Rokelle Lerner Associates
420 Summit Ave.
St. Paul, MN 55102
(612) 227-4031
writer, therapist, workshop leader

Jerry Moe
Sierra Tucson
16500 N. Lago del Oro
Tucson, AZ 85737-94062
(800) 624-9001
Director, Children's Program, writer

Sharon Wegscheider-Cruse and Joe Cruse, M.D.
Onsite Training and Consulting Inc.
2820 W. Main
Rapid City, SD 57702
(605) 341-7432
writers, trainers, treatment directors

Organizations

American Association for Therapeutic Humor
9040 Forstview Rd.
Skokie, IL 60203-1913
(312) 679-2593

Healing Through Laughter and Play Conferences
Institute for the Advancement of Human Behavior
P.O. Box 7226
Stanford, CA 94309
(415) 851-8411

New Directions Counseling Center
8140 N. Mopac, Bldg. 2, Suite 230
Austin, TX 78759-8860
(512) 343-9496 (Tobin's number)

Playmakers
P.O. Box 90488
Austin, TX 78709
(512) 346-7529 (Catalog, Toy-of-the-Month Club, etc.)

Project Adventure, Inc.
P.O. Box 100
Hamilton, MA 01936
(508) 468-7981

Synergy Counseling and Consulting
11940 Jollyville Rd., Suite 220 N
Austin, TX 78759
(512) 335-1123 (Tom's number)

Recovery Groups

Alcoholics Anonymous
Al-Anon
Adult Children of Alcoholics
Co-dependents Anonymous
Narcotics Anonymous
Overeaters Anonymous

and many others:
See local phone directory.

RESOURCE B

Publications

Playful Activities and Exercises

"New Games"

The New Games Book, Andrew Fluegelman, ed., Doubleday & Co., 1976

More New Games, Andrew Fluegelman, Doubleday & Co., 1981

New Games for the Whole Family, Dale N. LeFevre, Perigee Books, 1988

Playfair: Everybody's Guide to Non-competitive Games, Matt Weinstein and Joel Goodman, Impact Publishers, 1980

Initiative Games

The Bottomless Bag, Karl Rohnke, Kendall/Hunt, 1991

Cow's Tails and Cobras, Karl Rohnke, Project Adventure, 1977

Silver Bullets, Karl Rohnke, Project Adventure, 1984 (Contact Project Adventure for a catalog of its equipment and other valuable publications.)

Games for Schools and Educational Settings

The Cooperative Sports and Games Book, Terry Orlick, Pantheon Books, 1978

The Second Cooperative Sports and Games Book, Terry Orlick, Pantheon Books, 1982

100 Ways to Enhance Self-Concept in the Classroom, Jack Canfield and Harold Wells, Prentice Hall, 1976

General Merriment

The entire, ever-expanding library of Klutz books by John Cassidy and friends. Whether it is for juggling, magic, cooking, kooshing, harmonica-playing or more, there is a delightful recipe in each one for fun. Get 'em all!

The Flying Apparatus Catalog from Klutz Press, 2121 Staunton Ct., Palo Alto, CA 94306. A blend of unique, useless, and unbelievable goodies for those with unusual tastes in toys (like us). Especially recommended for neophyte jugglers.

HUMOResources Catalog from The HUMOR Project (see Joel Goodman in the previous list) is a unique collection of humorous books, periodicals, and tapes that will tickle your funnybone and increase your creativity. Who knows, someday we may be in there! Check it out.

The Toy Book, Gil Asakawa and Leland Rucker, Alfred A. Knopf, 1991. A wonderful guide to the toys and games of the baby-boomer generation. Highly recommended!

General Interest Books and Periodicals about Play

Beyond Boredom and Anxiety, Mihaly Csikszentmihalyi, Jossey-Bass, 1975

The Complete Juggler, Dave Finnigan, Vintage Books, 1987

Flow: The Psychology of Optimal Experience, Mihaly Csikszentmihalyi, Harper and Row, 1990

Growing Young, Ashley Montagu, Greenwood Publishing Group, 1989 (Call (203) 226-3571 for orders)

Healthy Pleasures, Robert Ornstein and David Sobel, Addison-Wesley, 1989

Homo Ludens, Johan Huizinga, Beacon Press, 1955

How to Play with Your Children, Brian and Shirley Sutton-Smith, Hawthorne Books, 1974

Lateral Thinking: Creativity Step by Step, Edward de Bono, Harper and Row, 1970

The Magical Child, Joseph Chilton Pearce, Bantam New Age Books, 1981

Play and Learning, Edited by Brian Sutton-Smith, Gardener Press, 1979

The Power of Play, Frank and Theresa Caplan, Anchor Books, 1974

The Silent Pulse, George Leonard, E. P. Dutton, 1978

The Ultimate Athlete, George Leonard, Avon Books, 1977

The Well-Played Game, Bernard De Koven, Anchor Books, 1978

The Wonderful Father Book, Richard Mann, Turnbull and Willoughby Publishers, Inc., 1985

Work, Play, and Type: Achieving Balance in Your Life, Judith A. Provost, Consulting Psychologists Press, 1990

You Don't Have to Go Home from Work Exhausted!, Ann McGee-Cooper, et al., Bowen and Rogers, 1990

Healing Through Laughter, Play, and Inner Work

A Book of Games: A Course in Spiritual Play, Hugh Prather, Doubleday & Co., Inc., 1981

A Journey Through Your Childhood, Christopher Biffle, Jeremy P. Tarcher, 1989

Anatomy of an Illness, Norman Cousins, Bantam Books, 1983

At a Journal Workshop, Ira Progoff, Dialogue House, 1975

Crazy Wisdom, Wes "Scoop" Nisker, Ten Speed Press, 1990

Focusing, Eugene Gendlin, Bantam Books, 1981

Getting Well Again, Stephanie Matthews-Simonton, O. Carl Simonton, and James L. Creighton, Bantam Books, 1978

Head First, Norman Cousins, E. P. Dutton, 1989

The Healing Power of Humor, Allen Klein, Jeremy P. Tarcher, 1989

Homecoming: Reclaiming and Championing Your Inner Child, John Bradshaw, Bantam Books, 1990

The Inner Image: A Resource for Type Development, William Yabroff, Consulting Psychologists Press, 1990

It's Never Too Late to Have a Happy Childhood, Claudia Black, Ballantine Books, 1989

It Will Never Happen to Me, Claudia Black, Ballantine Books, 1987

Kids' Power: Healing Games for Children of Alcoholics, Jerry Moe and Don Pohlman, Health Communications, 1989

The Laughter Prescription, Laurence J. Peter and Bill Dana, Ballantine Books, 1982

Learning to Love Yourself, Sharon Wegscheider-Cruse, Health Communications, 1987

Love, Medicine, and Miracles, Bernie S. Siegel, Harper and Row, 1986

Mind as Healer, Mind as Slayer, Kenneth Pelletier, Dell Books, 1977

The Miracle of Recovery, Sharon Wegscheider-Cruse, Health Communications, 1989

The Possible Human, Jean Houston, Jeremy P. Tarcher, 1982

The Power of Your Other Hand, Lucia Capacchione, Newcastle Publishing Company, 1988

Psychosynthesis, Roberto Assagioli, Penguin Books, 1971

Recovery of Your Inner Child, Lucia Capacchione, Simon and Schuster, 1991

Releasing, Patricia Carrington, William Morrow and Co., 1984

What We May Be, Piero Ferrucci, Jeremy P. Tarcher, 1982

Windows To Our Children, Violet Oaklander, Gestalt Journal, 1989

INDEX

275

ABOUT
THE
AUTHORS

TOBIN QUEREAU, M.A., L.P.C., is the Division Chairperson for Human Resource Development at Austin Community College, Austin, Texas. In addition to teaching in the Human Development and Human Services Departments of the college, he heads its Alcoholism and Substance Abuse Program. Tobin is also a Licensed Professional Counselor and a Certified Chemical Dependency Specialist with a private practice at New Directions Counseling Center, in Austin, where he works with individuals and couples and leads groups for Adult Children of Alcoholics.

A former preschool teacher, Tobin currently serves on the Board of the Texas Association for Children of Alcoholics, and is an active presenter of workshops and trainings in the fields of recovery, stress management, creativity, and leadership. He delights in writing, has been known to teach juggling (to neophytes only), and enjoys rowing when he can no longer avoid exercising.

TOM ZIMMERMANN, M.A., L.P.C., is a nationally known speaker on topics of health, humor, stress management, and team-building. A member of the National Speakers Association, he has a full schedule of engagements making presentations to businesses, schools, human service agencies, and the public on improving attitudes, interaction, and motivation.

A "recovering" teacher and counselor, once active in

public school settings, Tom is now a Licensed Professional Counselor with a private practice at Synergy Counseling and Consulting, in Austin. There he sees individuals, couples, and families and leads groups. Tom is a practitioner of Aikido, which he often blends into his presentations in unexpected and enlightening ways. His most enjoyable pastime is leading New Game Plan for Recovery workshops.